# Oklahoma Notes

Basic-Sciences Review for Medical Licensure
Developed at
The University of Oklahoma at Oklahoma City, College of Medicine

Suitable Reviews for:
National Board of Medical Examiners (NBME), Part I
Medical Sciences Knowledge Profile (MSKP)
Foreign Medical Graduate Examination in the Medical Sciences (FMGEMS)

# Oklahoma Notes

# *Histology*

Daniel L. Feeback

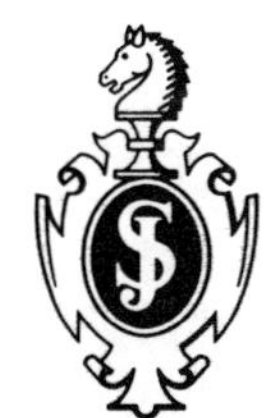

Springer-Verlag
New York Berlin Heidelberg
London Paris Tokyo

Daniel L. Feeback, Ph.D.
Department of Anatomical Sciences
Health Sciences Center
The University of Oklahoma at Oklahoma City
Oklahoma City, OK 73190
U.S.A.

Library of Congress Cataloging in Publication Data
Feeback, Daniel L.
Histology.
(Oklahoma notes)
1. Histology—Outlines, syllabi, etc. 2. Histology
—Examinations, questions, etc. I. Title. II. Series.
QM553.F45 1986 611′.018 86-26152



Copyrights and Acknowledgments begin on page 193, which constitutes a continuation of the copyright page.

Printed and bound by Quinn-Woodbine Inc., Woodbine, New Jersey.
Printed in the United States of America.

9 8 7 6 5 4 3 2 1

ISBN 0-387-96339-1 Springer-Verlag New York Berlin Heidelberg
ISBN 3-540-96339-1 Springer-Verlag Berlin Heidelberg New York

*To*
*Cynthia Ann*
*and*
*Shauna Lee*
*with love*

# Preface to the Oklahoma Notes

In 1973, the University of Oklahoma College of Medicine instituted a requirement for passage of the Part I National Boards for promotion to the third year. To assist students in preparation for this examination, a two-week review of the basic sciences was added to the curriculum in 1975. Ten review texts were written by the faculty: four in anatomical sciences and one each in the other six basic sciences. Self-instructional quizzes were also developed by each discipline and administered during the review period.

The first year the course was instituted the Total Score performance on National Boards Part I increased 60 points, with the relative standing of the school changing from 56th to 9th in the nation. The performance of the class has remained near the national candidate mean (500) since then, with a mean over the 12 years of 502 and a range of 467 to 537. This improvement in our own students' performance has been documented (Hyde et al: Performance on NBME Part I examination in relation to policies regarding use of test. J. Med. Educ. 60:439–443, 1985).

A questionnaire was administered to one of the classes after they had completed the boards; 82% rated the review books as the most beneficial part of the course. These texts have been recently updated and rewritten and are now available for use by all students of medicine who are preparing for comprehensive examinations in the Basic Medical Sciences.

RICHARD M. HYDE, Ph.D.
Executive Editor

## PREFACE

Preparation of a text intended largely for review of material to which students have been previously exposed through a formal course requires certain considerations and compromises. By nature, effective review books are shorter in length and less comprehensive in scope than texts utilized as course adjuncts. The reduction of a large body of information for review purposes should be one of selective condensation and not one of global, random deletion so that content remains significant and relevant. To be most useful, a review text should not be so general that it becomes ineffective and at the same time not so detailed that it represents an additional exhaustive treatise. Additionally, continuity and coherence must be maintained within the abbreviated format allowed. This work fulfills those criteria.

Histology or microanatomy, as an individual subject, is an amalgamation of many different but related disciplines including cytology, microscopic morphology, developmental microstructure, molecular biology, cellular genetics and physiology. As such, it encompasses an immense information base, some of which is repeated and hopefully reinforced in other courses of study. This text does not attempt in any way to cover all of these facets because realistically such an approach is not necessary to fulfill the role for which it is intended. Students of medicine, dentistry, veterinary science, mammalian biology and various allied health fields will find this book helpful in reviewing information to which they have been previously subjected in the context of conventional courses. Additionally, it will serve as an effective but time-conserving study guide for students of various disciplines preparing to sit for standardized proficiency examinations in which the basic science of histology is a component.

**D.L.F.**

## ACKNOWLEDGEMENTS

I would like to thank the many special people who have helped in the production of this book. It is gratifying to work with talented people and to be able to combine the fruits of their individual creative skills into a final product. I would particularly like to express my thanks to the artists who created the drawings that grace these pages. Artistic contributions were made by Dr. John W. Campbell, Phyllis L. Dillard, Laurie Forman Swaim, Shawn Schlinke and Evelyn Rullman. Special gratitude is extended to Ben Barnabas Han Soo Kew whose darkroom wizardry is responsible for each and every graphic reproduction of the artwork. His continuous reach for perfection, infinite attention to detail and perspicuous insight proved invaluable. I would like to acknowledge the scholarly contributions of Dr. Ronald Shew to the discussions of cartilaginous and osseous tissues, bone structure and bone growth. His expert knowledge of these subjects provided perceptive clarity to an otherwise complex area. Special accolades are due Pat Campbell who spent considerable effort and time in the tedious task of proofreading portions of the manuscript in its formative and final stages. To all of these exceptional people whose combined efforts augmented this endeavor, I am indebted.

# TABLE OF CONTENTS

# UNIT I: CELLS

Certain fundamental characteristics are common to all cells of the human organism. This is an expected occurrence since all such cells are descendants of a single cell, the zygote or fertilized ovum. The general features of a cell allow the observer to distinguish it as such while the cell's special characteristics, derived by differentiation from its progenitors, make classification into specific cell types possible. Comparatively, cells representing all parts of the human body tend to vary in more ways than they are similar. More importantly, the special morphologic and physiologic features of the differentiated cell correlates well with its functional role. Conversely, it is possible to make an educated prediction of the structural specializations required by a cell in order for it to carry out a specific physiologic function. Biologic systems are notoriously efficient and economical. Cells, representing true microcosms of biochemical activity, rarely possess organelles or chemical mediators unnecessary to fulfill their prescribed role.

Being able to recognize and categorize cells and the tissues and organs that they comprise as well as understanding the histophysiologic correlation between a structure and its function is the basis of medical histology. As such it forms the core for understanding and correlating alterations of structure and function basic to disease processes.

## HISTOLOGIC STAINING OF CELLS AND TISSUES

In order to visualize tissues and the cells that comprise them, it is necessary to use certain compounds capable of dyeing cellular components. Some of these are able to stain living cells and are referred to as supravital stains. More commonly in histologic preparations the cells and tissues have been treated to prevent subsequent loss of morphologic quality usually by treatment with solutions known collectively as fixatives. The cells in fixed tissues are dead but their morphology is preserved at the time of fixation. Many, but not all, fixatives work by altering certain constituents of the tissue such as denaturation of structural proteins. The most commonly used such fixative is an aqueous solution of formaldehyde referred to as formalin. Most tissues fix well when treated by submersion into 5% formalin buffered to near pH 7.0.

There are literally hundreds of dye chemicals capable of staining tissues various colors. The technique of choice for most routine work is the combined hematoxylin and eosin method (H&E). This procedure produces various shades of blue and pink for different reasons. Hematoxylin has an affinity for nucleic acids through a mechanism that is not entirely understood. In most methods DNA and RNA are stained blue. Eosin, on the other hand, works by a less complex and therefore better defined mechanism. The functional component of the dye is a colored anion, eosinate. It has a net negative charge and tends to bind to tissue and cellular components with positive charges through a process of simple dye-binding. In practice, blue or bluish structures usually indicate the presence of nucleic acids or acidic proteins and are designated as "hematoxylinophilic or basophilic" while other components are represented by shades of pink (referred to as "eosinophilic or acidophilic") or remain unstained ("neutrophilic"). It is noteworthy that most lipids are lost (dissolved out) in the processing of the tissue before staining and therefore are not available for staining in routinely prepared slides.

## THE TYPICAL CELL

It is helpful in studying the structure of cells to first note the component parts that are common to most cells followed by a study of the unusual structures that are found only in cells with a specialized function. The following structures, many of which are referred to as cellular organelles, will with few exceptions be present in all cells.

### Plasma Membrane

Key points concerning the plasma membrane (plasmalemma) include:

1) The plasma membrane can not be visualized directly by light microscopy but can be inferred by the smooth interface between free cells and their extracellular environment.

2) By electron microscopy the plasma membrane appears as a pair of electron-dense lines separated by a lucent space. For this reason it is sometimes referred to as a trilaminar membrane.

3) Usual width is approximately 8 nm. (Range: 7.5-10.0 nm).

4) Composition includes: (a) lipids, mostly phospholipids with smaller amounts of cholesterol, (b) proteins and (c) carbohydrates.

5) Current concepts based on biochemical assays and physical data such as freeze-fracture-etch studies indicate that the plasma membrane is composed of a phospholipid bilayer with each layer consisting of a

## MAJOR CELLULAR COMPONENTS

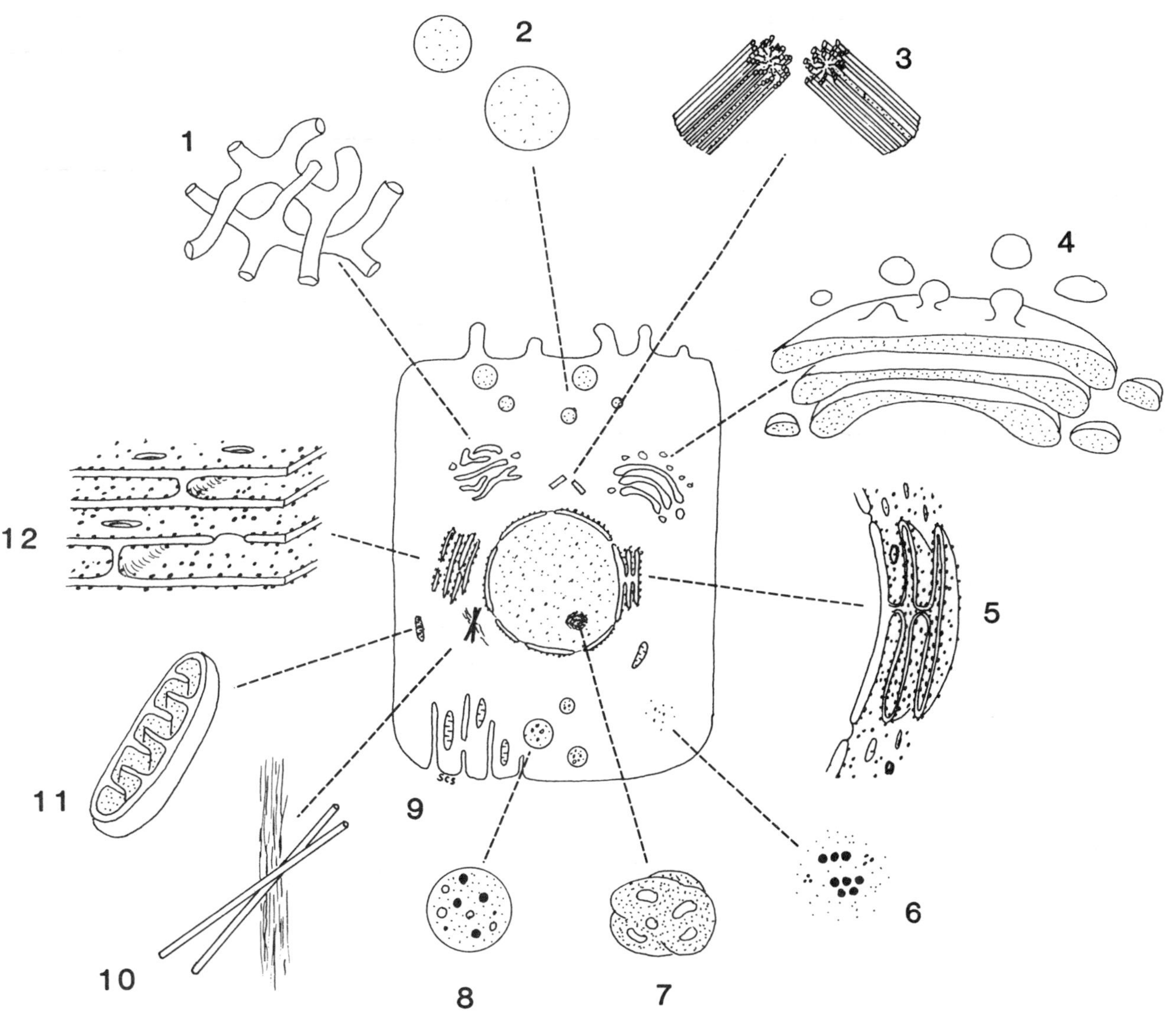


1: Smooth endoplasmic reticulum
2: Secretory granules
3: Centrioles (Diplosome)
4: Golgi apparatus
5: External face of nuclear envelope
6: Free ribosomes and glycogen granules
7: Nucleolus with nucleolonema
8: Lysosome
9: Basal infoldings with mitochondria
10: Microtubules and microfilaments
11: Mitochondrion
12: Rough endoplasmic reticulum

**Fig. 1.1.** Morphology of major cellular components.

hydrophobic end (linear tail) and a hydrophilic end (bulbous head). The hydrophobic tails of each layer project inward toward the center of the membrane while the hydrophilic ends are directed outward so that they interface with the external environment and the internal cellular milieu. Many of the membrane proteins are present as globular molecules intercalated among the lipid molecules. Their classification depends on whether they are bound to lipids (integral) or are less firmly associated with the lipid bimolecular layer (peripheral). The globular proteins may project from either surface of the membrane or pass completely through it (transmembranous). Some proteins may possess lipid (lipoproteins) or carbohydrate (glycoproteins) moieties. Some of the lipids may also bear carbohydrate side chains (glycolipids). The carbohydrate components project from the external surface of the plasma membrane where they are involved with cellular recognition, adhesion and binding of various molecules. Surface glycoproteins as well as poly- and oligosaccharides are present to some degree on all cells and are collectively referred to as the glycocalyx.

6) The plasma membrane delimits the outer boundaries of the cell and serves as a semipermeable barrier. Enzymes embedded within the membrane can also direct the flow of ions and molecules across the barrier with expenditure of energy (active transport).

## Ribosomes

Ribosomes are essential for synthesis of proteins either for export (secretion) or for internal use (structural proteins, enzymes). Important features of these structures include:

1) Ribosomes assemble amino acids into proteins as translated from messenger RNA (mRNA).

2) Ribosomes can not be seen by light microscopy but when present in abundance they impart basophilia to the cytoplasm due to the their content of ribonucleic acid.

3) Cells that synthesize protein in large quantities contain proportionately greater numbers of ribosomes.

4) With the resolution of the electron microscope, ribosomes are visualized directly as either free within the cytoplasm or attached to membranes. They are electron dense and measure 15-20 nm in diameter.

5) Ribosomes are composed of ribosomal RNA (rRNA) bound to protein and consist of two subunits (60S and 40S) which are synthesized within the nucleolus.

6) Polyribosomes (polysomes) are aggregates of ribosomes held together by a single strand of mRNA. They are often attached to cytoplasmic membranes but may be free within the cytoplasm as well.

## Endoplasmic Reticulum

The endoplasmic reticulum is a series of membranous structures and is present in two forms with differences in morphologic appearance and functional roles.

1) Rough (granular) endoplasmic reticulum (RER).
   a) The RER appears ultrastructurally as a series of parallel stacks of flattened cisternae with ribosomes attached to their surfaces.
   b) Abundant RER accounts for cytoplasmic basophilia at the light microscopic level.
   c) Quantity of RER correlates with protein synthetic activity of the cell.

2) Smooth (agranular) endoplasmic reticulum (SER).
   a) Cisternae are more tubular than flat and there are no associated ribosomes.
   b) Continuous with the RER.
   c) Responsible site for steroid synthesis, glycogen synthesis and conjugation, oxidation and methylation processes. Also is involved in contraction process of muscle cells as a specialized form, the sarcoplasmic reticulum.

## Golgi Apparatus

The Golgi apparatus is present in the vast majority of cells and appears as a series of stacked, flat saccules or cisternae exhibiting peripheral dilatations. The cisternae are all slightly curved producing a convex face (cis side or forming face) and a concave side (trans side or maturing face). Because of its function, it is best represented in cells which are largely secretory in nature. It can be visualized at the light microscopic level by use of special techniques and can be seen in some cells as a perinuclear clear area by routine staining methods. Its chief roles are:

1) Concentration and packaging of secretory components into membrane-bound secretory vesicles.

2) Glycosylation and sulfation of glycoproteins and glycolipids.

3) Proteolysis of presecretory proteins.

## Lysosomes

These are membrane-bound bodies that are morphologically heterogeneous. They are mostly spherical, electron-dense structures varying in size from 0.2 to 0.5 microns in diameter. They contain a variety of lytic enzymes. Most of these enzymes are active only at unphysiologic (acidic) hydrogen ion concentrations. Acid phosphatase serves as a histochemical marker for lysosomes. Their main role is the intracellular digestion of senescent organelles and phagocytosed material and in the metabolism of certain substances such as glycogen, cerebrosides, gangliosides, sphingomyelin and others.

1) Degradation of cytoplasmic organelles (autophagy).
   a) Organelles or portions of cytoplasm become membrane-bound (autophagic vacuole).
   b) Primary lysosomes fuse with the autophagic vacuole to form an autophagosome.
   c) Most hydrolyzed products are recycled but undigestible material may remain as residual bodies which may then be released extracellularly or accumulate intracellularly as lipofuscin (age) pigment.

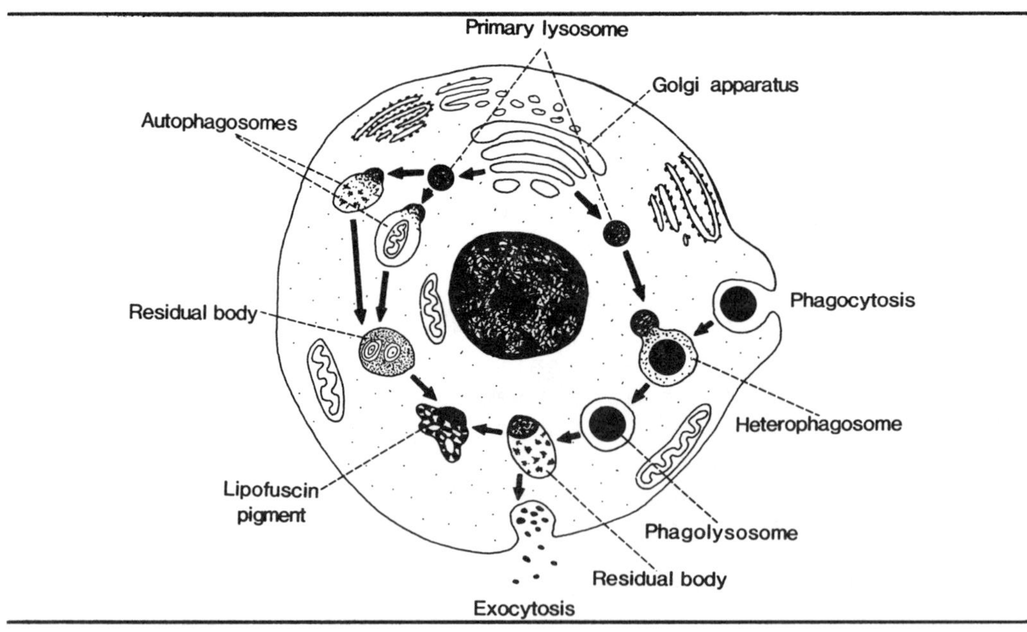


**Fig. 1.2.** The vacuolar system of a cell.

2) Degradation of extracellular (phagocytosed) material (heterophagy).

a) Phagocytosis results in intracytoplasmic membrane-bound bodies known as phagosomes (heterophagosomes).
b) Fusion with a primary lysosome results in formation of a secondary lysosome (phagolysosome).
c) Nondegradable substances appear as residual bodies which may be extruded through fusion with the plasmalemma (exocytosis) or remain within the cytoplasm.

3) Multivesicular bodies possibly represent another type of secondary lysosome that has the appearance of a membrane-bound vesicle containing acid hydrolases and other smaller membrane-bound vesicles. In some cases, the smaller vesicles may represent pincytotic vesicles.

## Peroxisomes

Peroxisomes (microbodies) are similar in size and appearance to lysosomes. They contain catalase which is capable of breaking down hydrogen peroxide formed from superoxide free radicals to water and oxygen. Their main role in man appears to be catabolism of hydrogen peroxide and superoxide anions which are extremely toxic to cells.

## Mitochondria

Mitochondria are very important organelles in that they serve as a major site of energy production through a variety of enzymes. They can produce high energy phosphorylated compounds (ATP) through the process of oxidative phosphorylation and are the site of the Krebs cycle enzymes. In addition to generating energy for the cell they also are capable of storing calcium as calcium phosphate granules (dense granules) within their matrix for subsequent release to the cell as the need arises. Although quite small, spheroid to ovoid structures (0.2 microns by up to 10 microns), they can often be visualized directly by phase contrast microscopy or by use of special staining techniques. Other points of importance include:

1) Delimited by a smooth outer membrane (external mitochondrial membrane) and an inner membrane (internal mitochondrial membrane) which is convoluted into a series of plicae (cristae). The cristae may appear flattened or tubular. The surface of the cristae facing the interior of the mitochondrion is covered focally by elementary particles which have a "lollipop-like" appearance ultrastructurally. The area of the mitochondrion enclosed by the internal mitochondrial membrane is termed the matrix.
   a) Respiratory chain enzymes (cytochromes, flavoproteins, dehydrogenases) reside on the

internal mitochondrial membrane.

b) Enzymes of oxidative phosphorylation and ATPase are located within the elementary particles.

c) Krebs cycle enzymes are located within the matrix.

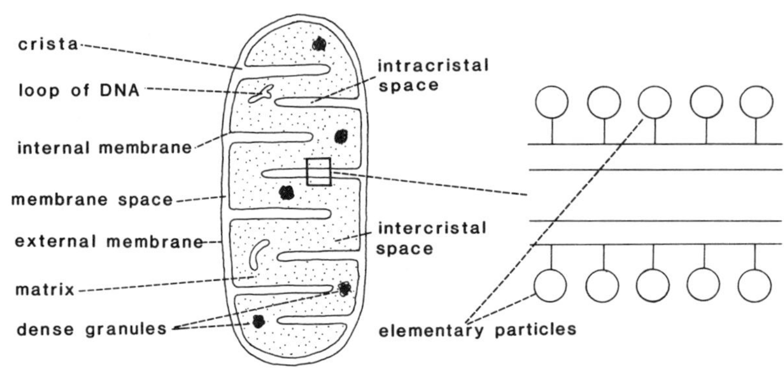


**Fig. 1.3.** Ultrastructure of a mitochondrion. (Courtesy Dr. R. Snell.)

2) Mitochondria are motile and can be seen to move within the cytoplasm.

3) They are capable of self replication through a budding process and contain their own DNA, RNA and ribosomes within the matrix enabling synthesis of proteins.

## Cytoskeletal Elements

The cytoskeletal elements maintain control of cellular shape and are important in cellular motility and division. There are several types of structures that fall into this category including microtubules and various sizes of filaments. Key points include:

1) Cytoskeletal elements can not be resolved at the light microscopic level unless present in thick bundles (fibrils).

2) Microtubules are thin (25 nm diameter) hollow tubes (15 nm lumen) which vary in length up to several microns.

a) Composed of the protein, tubulin, present as dimers that are organized into a helix of protofilaments.

b) They are very labile structures which change length by polymerization and depolymerization.

c) Microtubules are involved in movement of

chromosomes during mitosis and are integral components of other organelles such as centrioles, basal bodies, cilia and flagella.

3) Filamentous cytoskeletal elements include microfilaments, intermediate filaments and thick filaments.
   a) Microfilaments (6 nm thick) are present mostly as actin. Actin is a major contractile protein in muscle cells but is found in varying amounts in all cells. Another important microfilament is spectrin, which may link actin to plasma membrane proteins.
   b) Intermediate filaments (8-10 nm thick) so named because they are intermediate in size between thick and microfilaments include a diversity of filament types. They do not seem to be contractile in nature but provide three-dimensional support for the cell. They include:

      i) Tonofilaments (prekeratin) within epithelial cells.
      ii) Neurofilaments within certain neurons.
      iii) Glial filaments (glial fibrillary acidic protein) within astrocytes.
      iv) Desmin filaments primarily within certain muscle cells.
      v) Vimentin within mesenchymal or mesenchymally-derived cells.

   c) Thick filaments (15 nm thick) consist of myosin, the other major contractile protein of muscle cells. They are present in many nonmuscle cells as well.

## Centrioles

Centrioles are cylindrical bodies composed of nine sets of triplet microtubules. They occur in pairs (diplosomes) near the center of the cell and are oriented with their long axes at right angles to each other. They measure about 150 nm in diameter and 300-500 nm in length. Centrioles play a key role in cellular division and are capable of reproducing themselves as well as producing structurally identical basal bodies which form the base of cilia. Centrioles are absent from some highly-differentiated cells which consequently lose the ability to reproduce. Examples include neurons and cardiac muscle cells.

## Cytoplasmic Inclusions

Individually, inclusions unlike most organelles are variably present within the cellular cytoplasm. However, most cells usually possess one or more types of inclusions while some cells harbor specific types related to their function.

1) Pigments.
   a) Melanin is present in skin and hair cells, pigment epithelial cells of the eye, and the meninges of the brain. Neuromelanin which differs biochemically from melanin is present within certain neurons of the central nervous system.
   b) Lipofuscin is a golden-brown, membrane-bound pigment associated with lysosomal activity. It is most abundant in aged post-mitotic cells such as cardiac muscle cells and neurons.

2) Glycogen is a carbohydrate (polymerized glucose molecules) that is stored within the cytoplasm of many cell types. It can be demonstrated in cells and tissues fixed with appropriate nonaqueous solutions and then stained with the periodic acid-Schiff (PAS) technique which imparts a magenta color to glycogen containing sites. In electron micrographs glycogen appears as free electron-dense particles measuring 15-30 nm in diameter. Single particles are termed alpha particles while large aggregates (rosettes) are called beta particles.

3) Lipid droplets are not preserved in routine histologic preparation for light microscopy but if large enough create the appearance of clear spaces within the cells. Fat cells (lipocytes) which contain an enormous lipid droplet as their major cytoplasmic component appear to be empty. Under the electron microscope, lipid vacuoles appear as dark, round structures not enclosed by a membrane.

4) Membrane-bound secretory granules (vesicles) are transiently present in cells which function in secretion of protein or mucin for extracellular transport.

5) Coated vesicles are often found in cells active in endocytosis of extracellular macromolecules. They have the appearance under the electron microscope of vesicles sparsely coated with stubby bristles extending outward into the cytosol. Special techniques have disclosed the three-dimensional structure as a polygonal meshwork of material applied to the outer surface of the vesicle membrane. The composition of the coat has been shown to be largely a protein called clathrin.

6) Crystals (crystalloids) are present in certain cells including the Leydig and Sertoli cells of the testes.

They are apparently protein in nature and of unknown functional significance.

## Nucleus

The nucleus is the most visibly conspicuous structure within the cell. It is enclosed by a nuclear envelope and contains dispersed strands of DNA (chromatin) and one or more nucleoli. Although most cells contain a single nucleus some cells are occasionally binucleate (some liver cells and urothelial cells). Skeletal muscle cells and osteoclasts are multinucleate.

1) Nuclear envelope.
   a) Consists of a pair of 7-8 nm thick membranes separated by a narrow (40-70 nm) perinuclear cisterna. The outer membrane is often studded with ribosomes and is continuous with the RER.
   b) Nuclear pores (70 nm in diameter), octagonal in shape and covered by a thin diaphragm, are present which allow nuclear-cytoplasmic exchange of small molecules including mRNA.

2) Chromatin.
   a) Composed of coiled strands of DNA bound to basic proteins (histones). Small particles visible with the electron microscope represent repeating units containing a core of histones. These units, called nucleosomes, are surrounded by DNA in a helical fashion that binds them together. The string of nucleosomes is then secondarily coiled into a superhelix which results in the appearance of a fibril at the electron microscopic level.
   b) Heterochromatin is stainable and visible by light microscopy. It represents an inactive form of condensed DNA. Inactivated X chromosomes (Barr bodies) and the chromosomes in actively dividing cells consist entirely of heterochromatin. In most cells, heterochromatin may be seen adhering to the nuclear envelope or adjacent to the nucleolus. It is quite electron-dense by electron microscopy.
   c) Euchromatin is not visualized directly by light microscopy but is evident by poorly stained areas between the heterochromatin. Electron micrographs reveal it as a loose network of fine fibrils (<u>vide supra</u>). It represents the active site of DNA transcription. The amount present is a rough indicator of the rate of transcription occurring within the nucleus.

3) Nucleolus.
   a) Each cell contains one or more nucleoli which

represent the site of mRNA synthesis.

b) It stains basophilic and is visible with the light microscope as a round to oval intranuclear structure.

c) There are two major components observed by electron microscopy:

   i) Pars fibrosa is composed of densely packed ribonucleoprotein filaments.
   
   ii) Pars granulosa (nucleolonema) consists of ribonucleoprotein particles.

## CELLULAR DIFFERENTIATION AND FUNCTIONAL SPECIALIZATION

In order to perform their various functions and best cope with their environment, cells are capable of acquiring a variety of morphologic and biochemical characteristics through a process of genetically controlled differentiation. An organized approach to the study of cellular functional adaptations is best effected by examining the structural modifications that may be observed at the level of individual cellular organelles. Structural modifications can then be related to the physiologic role of the individual cells that possess them.

### Specializations of the Plasma Membrane

Many of the structural modifications of the plasma membrane are to be found on the surfaces of epithelial cells and as such are referred to as "surface modifications". In these cells, they provide a variety of specialized functions including mechanical or chemical protection, absorption, secretion, excretion, movement of cells or surface substances and reception of external stimuli. It is convenient to study these in association with their location on the surface of the cell. They may occur on lateral, basal and apical surfaces. Structural alterations of the plasma membrane are not, however, limited to epithelial cells.

#### Lateral Surface Specializations

Most lateral cell surface specializations are classified as junctions, which aid in the binding of cells together and in special cases, allow cell-to-cell communication. Junctional complexes are lateral border modifications in which several specific types of junctions function together. The major types of junctions include:

1) Zonula occludens (occluding junction).

   a) In this type, the outer leaflet of the plasma membrane is shared by two adjacent cells in a band-like (zonula) pattern most often associated with the lateral apical aspects of the two cells. Many cells can then participate in this type of junction to effectively prevent substances from entering between the cells from their apices along their lateral borders.

b) Occluding junctions do not possess much inherent mechanical strength and are therefore easily disrupted by mechanical forces if not reinforced by other types of cell junctions.

2) Zonula adherens (adhering junction).

a) Appears as a thickening in the inner leaflet of the plasma membrane. May often be found just below the zonula occludens. Filaments are associated with this type which reinforce the junction by dispersing the strain from the site of membrane binding.

b) Zonula adherens is often found just below the zonula occludens where it aids in mechanical support of the occluding junction.

3) Macula adherens (desmosome).

a) Desmosomes are focal binding areas between cells (usually epithelial) subjected to mechanical stress. They have been compared to "spot welds" and are partially responsible for the intercellular bridges seen by light microscopy.

b) Ultrastructurally, the inner lamella of the plasma membrane in the macular area is associated with a dense, plaque-like thickening in which numerous filaments are embedded. The intercellular space in these regions is reduced and filled with an electron-dense granular material.

c) Desmosomes may be found alone or as part of a junctional complex.

4) Junctional complexes are responsible for the terminal bars seen at lateral apical cell boundaries of certain epithelial cells at the light microscopic level. From the apex toward the base along the lateral border of the cell, the junctional complex is seen to consist of zonula occludens, zonula adherens and macula adherens.

5) Communicating junctions.

a) Also known as a nexus, gap junction or macula communicans. In these the cell membranes of adjacent cells come into very close contact without fusion. They behave functionally as cellular synapses and are sites of cell-to-cell communication enabling integrated or coordinated responses.

b) This type of junction is very labile and may be lost and then reformed later. The intercalated disk of cardiac muscle fibers seen by light microscopy functions partially as a mechanical junction and partially as a communicating junction.

c) Gap junctions are difficult to demonstrate directly by electron microscopy but in areas of macular membrane approximation (within 2 nm) numerous bridging structures can be observed (connexons). With special transmission EM techniques, the connexon appears to be composed of a central annulus surrounded by six subunits.

Another type of lateral surface modification associated with junctions is the <u>bile canaliculus</u> present between apposing hepatocytes. Bile canaliculi are formed by serpentine indentions of the plasma membranes of contiguous liver cells. Zonulae occludentes are found along the length of the canaliculi which effect an impermeable seal to separate bile flow from blood flow.

## <u>Basal Surface Specializations</u>

Cells that rest on connective tissue (most epithelia) usually sit directly on an intervening basement membrane. It is not truly a modification of the plasma membrane but is found in close apposition to the basal aspect of certain cell types. When subjected to mechanical forces they are often bound to this basement membrane by modified membrane-associated junctions known as hemidesmosomes.

1) Basement membrane.

a) The designation "basement membrane" refers to a structure observed first with the light microscope in tissues stained by silver impregnation or with the PAS method. When examination by the electron microscope became available it revealed that the originally described basement membrane beneath many epithelial cells was composed of two distinct components:

i) Amorphous basal lamina.

ii) Thin layer of reticular fibers, the lamina reticularis.

b) Both components are present beneath some epithelial cells while in certain areas (renal glomerulus, pulmonary alveoli and lens capsule) only a very thick basal lamina is present.

c) The basal lamina is composed of glycoproteins and Type IV collagen fibers. It lies just subjacent to the epithelial cells which are thought to secrete it. The reticular lamina lies just beneath the basal lamina and consists of reticular fibers embedded in a polysaccharide- and glycoprotein-containing matrix. It is believed to be elaborated by the underlying connective tissue.

2) Hemidesmosomes.
   a) These are another type of junction which unlike those found on lateral surfaces are asymmetrical.
   b) Similar in appearance to half a desmosome, they apparently serve to bind the cell base to its underlying basement membrane.

Another type of basal surface modification referred to as <u>basal striations</u> or infoldings appear as redundant invaginations in the basal plasma membrane of distal tubule cells in the kidney and the striated ductal cells of the major salivary glands. These along with longitudinally arranged rod-shaped mitochondria within the folds produce the striate appearance seen by optical microscopy. Such characteristics are associated with cells involved in active ion transport.

## Apical Surface Specializations

The free surface modifications associated with the plasma membrane of epithelial cells provide the cell with the structural format to perform their diverse roles. Certain cytoskeletal elements may be seen in association with the apical plasma membrane providing additional structural modifications and functional multiplicity.

1) Glycocalyx.
   a) Coats the plasma membrane of most cell types.
   b) Especially prominent on apical surfaces of absorptive cells of small intestine where it consists not only of glycoproteins but contains disaccharidases and alkaline phosphatase.
   c) Besides its known involvement in cell-to-cell adhesion, communication and recognition, it also provides a specialized site for various chemical reactions at the cell surface.

2) Microvilli.
   a) Present on the luminal surface of cells involved in absorption, they can be observed in aggregate but not individually with the light microscope producing a characteristic appearance. When associated with absoptive cells of the gastro-intestinal tract, the term <u>striate border</u> is applied. A similar structure observed on cells of the proximal tubule of the kidney is called the <u>brush border</u>.

b) The structures above result from regular, parallel evaginations of the plasma membrane and underlying cytoplasm extending from the surface of the cell. Each individual projection is a microvillus. They contain a 6 nm core of microfilaments (largely actin) arranged parallel to the long axis of the microvillus which attaches to the microvillar tip (dense tip) and at the basal position is intertwined with a dense meshwork of other filaments. This arrangement at the bases of contiguous microvilli produces a linear density running parallel to the apical surface of the cell. It is observable by optical microscopy as the terminal web.

c) Microvilli increase considerably the apical surface area of the cell enhancing its absorptive efficiency.

3) Stereocilia.

a) Present on apical surfaces of principal cells lining the ductus epididymis and a portion of the ductus deferens.

b) Basic structure is similar to microvilli but stereocilia are larger, longer and frequently anastomose.

c) Stereocilia are not structurally or functionally related to cilia, the term is unfortunately misleading.

4) Cilia.

a) Cilia are plasma membrane-covered evaginations of the cell surface. They are motile and because many of them are present per cell, they can be resolved with the light microscope.

b) Typically, cilia measure 5-10 microns in length and 0.2 microns in diameter. They are cylindrical and covered externally by plasma membrane. There are two basic parts, the apical axoneme which protrudes above the surface of the cell and the basal body analogous in structure to the centriole from which it is derived.

i) The internal ultrastructure of the axoneme reveals a central pair of microtubules surrounded by nine peripheral doublets (axonemal 9+2 complex). The central doublet is enclosed within a sheath from which radial spokes extend and connect with the outer nine doublets. These are in turn connected peripherally by links composed of nexin. Outer and inner arms extend from each peripheral doublet toward the adjacent doublet. These arms are composed partially of dynein, the force-generating enzyme.

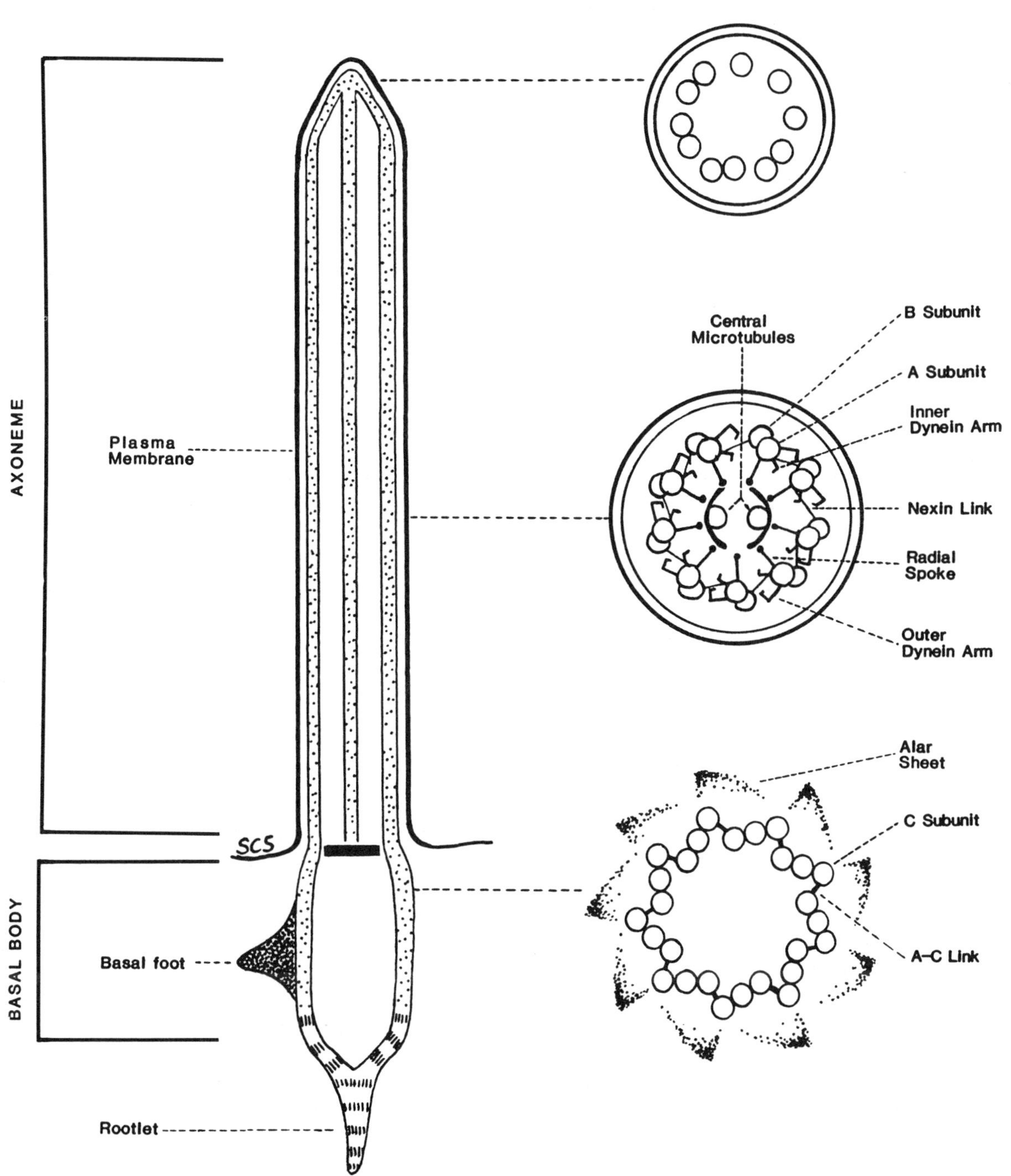


**Fig. 1.4.** Ultrastructure of a cilium and its basal body.

ii) The basal body, like its centriole progenitor, is composed of nine triplet microtubules. Fibrous material extends from the basal end of each triplet to form the rootlet which bears periodic cross-striations. A pyramidal basal foot is present oriented in the direction of the effective beat of the cilium.

c) Cilia are located in the respiratory tract (upper and lower) and within the fallopian tubes. They are important functionally in moving materials (mucous) or cells (ova, sperm) along an epithelial surface.

4) Flagella are restricted to the tail of spermatozoa in the human where one or two per sperm cell may be found. They are structurally similar to cilia but usually much longer.

## Special Plasma Membrane Modifications

Unusual modifications of the plasma membrane may be found associated with myelin producing cells of the nervous system and certain receptor (transducer) cells of special senses.

Both the oligodendroglia cell of the central nervous system and the Schwann cell of the peripheral nervous system are capable of myelinating nerve cell processes by the deposition of abundant compact, concentric layers of specialized plasma membrane around the neurite albeit by perhaps different mechanisms. In either case the membrane ensheathment results in insulating properties that increases the conduction velocity of the nerve impulse.

The photoreceptor cells of the retina (rods and cones) contain outer segments consisting of hundreds of uniform, membranous disks that are formed by repeated infoldings of the plasma membrane. Besides the redundant membranous folds, a typical basal body from which emanate nine doublet microtubules (the central pair is absent) connect the outer segments with the inner segments suggesting that the former are highly modified cilia. Associated with the membranes of the disks are visual pigments capable of converting photon energy into generator potentials. The enormous membrane surface increases the efficiency of photic absorption and transduction.

The hair cells of the maculae of the saccule and utricle and in the cristae ampullaris of the three semicircular canals of the inner ear bear a number of nonmotile microvilli (stereocilia) and a single true cilium (kinocilium). Deformation of the hair cells by linear acceleration or gravity induces the hair cells to produce a generator potential. Straight microvilli are present on the surface of the hair cells of the organ of Corti where vibratory energy along the basilar membrane causes deformation of the hair cells and subsequent production of a generator potential.

### Specializations of Cytoplasmic Organelles

For the most part, intracellular organelles do not undergo significant morphologic specialization. Instead, quantitative and locational adaptations of these components serve the needs of the specialized cell. For example, cells requiring large amounts of energy through oxidative metabolism will likely contain abundant mitochondria which are likely to be located proximate to the intracellular location where the high energy phosphorated compounds are required (basal striations of distal convoluted tubule cells of kidney nephron). Likewise, cells whose function is largely phagocytic in nature will contain numerous lysosomes (macrophages and certain granular leukocytes). On the other hand, organelles not necessary for the cell to carry out its specific function are not likely to be found in untoward amounts.

## THE CELL CYCLE AND CELL DYNAMICS

The life span of various cell types covers a wide temporal range related in part to their functional roles and degree of differentiation. Generally, cells gain functional specialization at the expense of proliferative capability. Certain cells belong to a population which requires constant renewal because of loss through normal attrition. Most epithelial cells fall into this category because loss of mature cells occurs at the interface of the epithelium with the external environment. These surface cells are usually those most specialized for their functional role but because of their degree of specialization they are incapable of maintaining the population through cellular division. This problem is solved by the presence of relatively undifferentiated cells which, though functionally inept, constantly contribute new cells which can subsequently differentiate into mature functional cells. Constantly renewing cells belong to a category collectively known as the labile cell population. This population includes, besides the cells composing various epithelia, certain connective tissues cells especially those that reside in reticular connective tissues.

In contrast to the labile cell population are other highly specialized cells which have completely reliquished the ability to proliferate and lack reserve cells able to divide and replace cells lost to age-related attrition or disease. These cells which include neurons and cardiac muscle cells are no longer capable of mitosis once their mature populations are established and reside in a so-called post-mitotic state. They belong to the permanent cell population.

Intermediate to these two categories are cells which normally do not require constant renewal but maintain a latent capacity for cell replacement which is expressed under conditions of demand. This cell population is known as the stable cell population and is typified by functional liver cells, the hepatocytes.

The concept of a cell cycle is based on the fact that certain cell types are known to divide over and over again at regular intervals. Cells enter the cycle at the time they are formed by the division of a progenitor cell and end their cycle upon their death or by dividing through a process known as mitosis to form two new daughter cells. Newly formed daughter cells may then enter their own cell cycle. From the discussion above it is obvious that not all cells are "in cycle". Cell populations that require constant renewal (labile cells) possess a number of relatively undifferentiated cells that are constantly cycling to meet the needs of the tissue which they comprise. Permanent cell populations have left the cycle completely and have no reserve cells capable of reentering it regardless of demand. These cell are permanently "out of cycle". Cells of the stable population are normally "out of cycle" but if the need arises they may resume cyclic activity.

The cell cycle is generally divided into two periods, a short but fairly constant one in terms of time, termed mitosis during which the cell is dividing and another longer but more highly variable one, occuring between mitotic divisions, known as interphase. Interphase is further subdivided into three phases. Based on light microscopic morphology, mitosis is said to consist of four consecutive phases. Certain highlights are worthy of review:

THE CELL CYCLE

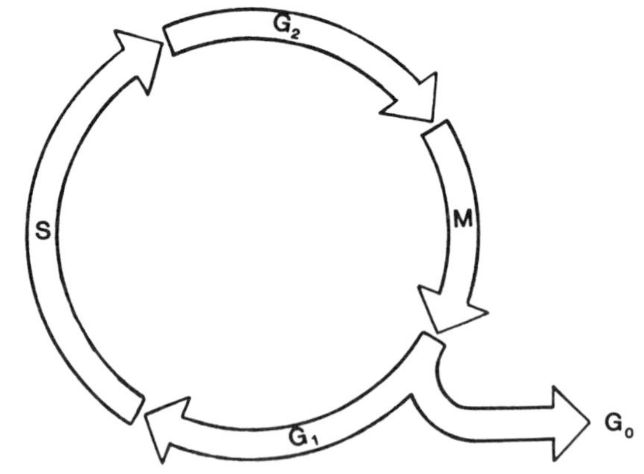


**Fig. 1.5.** Major intervals of the cell cycle.

1) The cell enters its cycle after mitotic division of its progenitor at the beginning of interphase which

includes:

a) $G_1$ (First gap), an interval of cell growth and protein synthesis. Specialized functions of cells are often performed in an extended $G_1$ phase.

b) S (DNA Synthesis), the interval in which DNA duplication occurs in preparation for mitosis.

c) $G_2$ (Second gap), an interval in which proteins which participate in cell division (such as tubulin) are synthesized and centriole replication occurs.

2) M (Mitosis) follows interphase and although dynamic and continuous it is divided into four morphologic phases:

a) <u>Prophase</u> is characterized by migration of the two pairs of centrioles to opposite poles, organization of microtubules into the mitotic spindle and the appearance of astral rays, loss of nuclear membrane and nucleolus and condensation of nuclear chromatin into thread-like structures corresponding to the 46 pairs of chromosomes.

b) <u>Metaphase</u> continues as further condensation of chromatin into distinct chromosomes that occupy the equitorial plane of the cell oriented at a right angle to the long axis of the mitotic spindle. Each of the 46 chromosome pairs is composed of two discrete structures (chromatids) attached to each other at a single point (centromere). Portions of the centromere (kinetochores) act as chromosomal microtubule organizing centers. Microtubules connect the chromatids at their centromere to the centrioles in opposite poles of the cell. The morphologic hallmark of metaphase is the point at which the centromeres of all 46 pairs of chromatids line up along the equitorial plane with separation of the chromatids along their length except at the point of centromeric union.

c) <u>Anaphase</u> commences with centromeric division and the concomitant appearance of 92 individual chromosomes which through a still obsure process half move to one cellular pole while the other half move to the opposite pole. Disassembly and reassembly of spindle tubulin and the interaction of actin and myosin may be involved in the process of movement.

d) <u>Telophase</u> is heralded by the reformation of nuclear membranes around each chromosome complement, followed by dispersion of chromosomes into thread-like chromatin, appearance of nucleoli and concomitant with these nuclear events (karyokinesis), cytoplasmic division (cytokinesis) occurs.

# MITOSIS

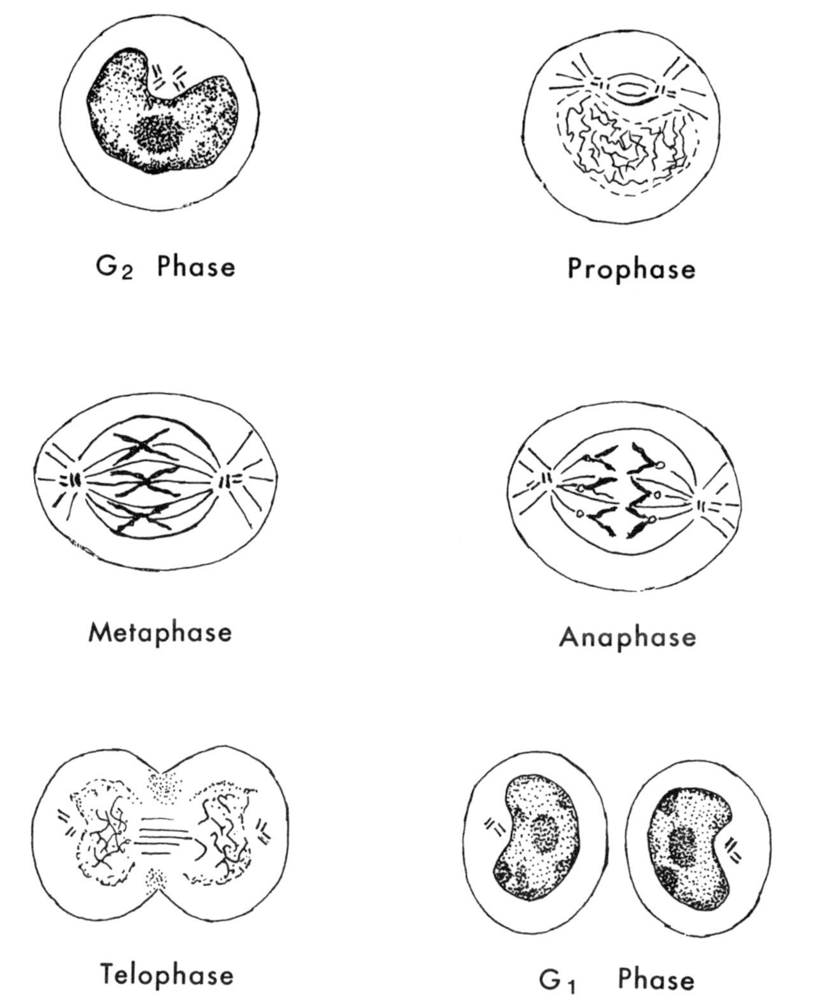


**Fig. 1.6.** Stages of mitosis and the $G_1$ and $G_2$ phases of interphase.

Cells comprising permanent cell populations lack a means of replacing lost cells and are outside of the cell cycle. Cells of the stable cell population are also "out of cycle", a condition which is indefinite in length but not necessarily permanent. Cells in this category are said to reside in the $G_0$ state. Constantly renewing cell populations (labile cells) contain a subpopulation of cells which are constantly cycling with all stages of the cell cycle represented at some point.

It should be noted that the germ cells (oogonia and spermatogonia) proliferate by mitosis while their differentiated cellular progeny (primary oocytes and spermatocytes) undergo a modified type of cellular division known as meiosis in which there is a final reduction of the chromosomal number to one-half (haploid) of the normal 46 chomosomal complement.

In the male, there are no primary spermatocytes produced until puberty. Once produced they can then enter meiotic division to produce mature spermatozoa. In the female, the primary oocytes develop in the fetus and enter meiosis where they are suspended within prophase of the first meiotic division. The primary oocytes do not complete the first meiotic division until after the onset of puberty and then only on an individual basis just before follicular rupture with monthly ovulation. The second meiotic division is not completed unless fertilization occurs.

## UNIT I: PROFICIENCY EXAM

**DIRECTIONS:** For the following questions select the one best answer which completes the statement or answers the question.

1) The hydrophobic linear tails of the phospholipid bilayer composing the plasma membrane:
   A. Are directed outward into the extracellular environment.
   B. Are directed inward into the cytosol.
   C. Are a component of the glycocalyx.
   D. Project inward into the interior of the membrane.
   E. Are solely responsible for the antigenic properties of the cell.

2) Polyribosomes are aggregates of ribosomes held together by:
   A. Van der Waals forces.
   B. Microfilaments.
   C. Linear strands of messenger RNA.
   D. Ionized sialic acid residues.
   E. Calmodulin.

3) A perinuclear clear area (Hof) in a cell with prominent cytoplasmic basophilia likely represents the intracytoplasmic location of:
   A. The Golgi apparatus.
   B. Terminal cisternae of granular endoplasmic reticulum.
   C. Centriolar replication.
   D. Zymogen granules.
   E. Aggregates of lipofuscin granules.

4) Which of the following organelles lacks a membranous component?
   A. Nuclear envelope.
   B. Lysosome.
   C. Mitochondrion.
   D. Glycogen rosette.
   E. Smooth endoplasmic reticulum.

5) Tonofilaments are:
   A. A type of intermediate filament.
   B. Composed of polymerized tubulin.
   C. Associated with the mitotic spindle.
   D. Located within the matrix of mitochondria.
   E. Smaller in diameter than actin filaments.

6) The morphologic characteristics of a cell involved in synthesis of large amounts of protein for export would include all the following EXCEPT:
   A. A well-developed Golgi apparatus.
   B. Prominent nucleoli.
   C. Abundant granular endoplasmic reticulum.
   D. Cytoplasmic basophilia.
   E. A nucleus containing a preponderance of heterochromatin.

7) Which of the following would NOT be found within a mitochondrion?
   A. Dense granules.
   B. RNA.
   C. DNA.
   D. Coated vesicles.
   E. Elementary particles.

8) Primary lysosomes contain:
   A. Numerous glycogen particles.
   B. Acid phosphatase.
   C. Catalase.
   D. Lipofuscin pigment.
   E. RNA.

9) Cells containing abundant lysosomes are likely to be specialized for:
   A. Contraction.
   B. Excitability.
   C. Secretion.
   D. Absorption.
   E. Phagocytosis.

10) A terminal web is associated with:
   A. Hemidesmosomes.
   B. The apical tip of the ciliary axoneme.
   C. The basal portion of the striate border.
   D. Desmosomes.
   E. None of the above.

11) The force-generating enzyme of a cilium is known as:
   A. Tubulin.
   B. Desmin.
   C. Myosin.
   D. Transmutin.
   E. Dynein.

12) Which of the following structures is greatest in length?
  A. Microvillus.
  B. Stereocilium.
  C. Cilium.
  D. Flagellum.
  E. Mitochondrion.

13) Centrioles are replicated in:
  A. The $G_1$ phase.
  B. Prophase.
  C. The nucleolus.
  D. Anaphase.
  E. The $G_2$ phase.

14) Which of the following can NOT be observed directly with the light microscope?
  A. Diplosome.
  B. Nucleolus.
  C. Heterochromatin.
  D. Plasma membrane.
  E. Cilia.

15) Replication of DNA in a normal mitotic division occurs in:
  A. Interphase.
  B. Prophase.
  C. Metaphase.
  D. Anaphase.
  E. Telophase.

**CHANGE IN FORMAT:** For the following questions select:

  (A) if only 1, 2 and 3 are correct.
  (B) if only 1 and 3 are correct.
  (C) if only 2 and 4 are correct.
  (D) if only 4 is correct.
  (E) if all are correct.

16) Which of the following are motile?
  1. Cilia.
  2. Mitochondria.
  3. Flagella.
  4. Stereocilia.

17) Which of the following are self-replicating?
  1. Lysosomes.
  2. Mitochondria.
  3. Microtubules.
  4. Centrioles.

**(A) = 1, 2, 3 (B) = 1, 3 (C) = 2, 4 (D) = 4 only (E) = All**

18) The junctional complex consists of which of the following?
   1. Zonula occludens.
   2. Zonula adherens.
   3. Macula adherens.
   4. Nexus.

19) The basal lamina contains:
   1. Type IV collagen.
   2. Reticular fibers.
   3. A glycoprotein known as laminin.
   4. Phospholipid.

20) Characteristics of steroid-producing cells include:
   1. Abundant smooth endoplasmic reticulum.
   2. Cytoplasmic lipid droplets.
   3. Mitochondria with tubular cristae.
   4. Numerous free ribosomes in the cytoplasm.

21) Enzymes of the Krebs cycle are located:
   1. On the internal mitochondrial membrane.
   2. Within the spherical portion of the elementary particles.
   3. On the outer mitochondrial membrane.
   4. Within the mitochondrial matrix.

22) Microtubules are integral components of:
   1. Centrioles.
   2. Basal bodies.
   3. Cilia.
   4. Flagella.

23) Intermediate filaments include:
   1. Actin filaments.
   2. Neurofilaments.
   3. Myosin filaments.
   4. Tonofilaments.

24) Ribosomes may be found attached to the surface of the:
   1. Outer nuclear membrane.
   2. Internal nuclear membrane.
   3. Endoplasmic reticulum.
   4. Mature face of the Golgi apparatus.

25) The glycocalyx functions in:
   1. Cell-to-cell adhesion.
   2. Molecular recognition.
   3. Chemical reactions.
   4. Cell-to-cell communication.

# UNIT II: TISSUES

Tissues are composed of cells and intercellular material produced mostly by the component cells. The cellular density and the amount and composition of extracellular matrix varies widely among different types of tissues. Tissues are specialized to carry out specific roles and are found not as individual units but rather together in various combinations as integral and functional components of organs and body parts. There are four basic tissue types found in the human body that can be further subdivided by differential features.

Tissues may be classified as:

1) Epithelial tissue
   a) Surfacing epithelia
   b) Secreting epithelia (glands)
   c) Special epithelia

2) Connective tissue
   a) Embryonal connective tissue
      i) Mesenchyme
      ii) Mucous connective tissue
   b) Adult connective tissue
      i) Connective tissue proper
         1) Areolar connective tissue
         2) Dense irregular connective tissue
         3) Dense regular connective tissue
         4) Other types
            a) Adipose connective tissue
            b) Fibrofatty connective tissue
            c) Pigmented connective tissue
            d) Elastic connective tissue
      ii) Special connective tissue
         1) Cartilaginous tissue
         2) Osseous (bony) tissue
         3) Reticular connective tissue

3) Muscular tissue
   a) Smooth muscle tissue
   b) Skeletal muscle tissue
   c) Cardiac muscle tissue

4) Nervous tissue

# EPITHELIAL TISSUES

Epithelia are defined as continuous unilaminar or multilaminar sheets of cells that cover a body surface. This surface may be external or internal and may be extensive or notable only at the microscopic level. Internal surfaces may be open to the external environment directly or indirectly or may form the boundaries of a closed cavity. In common, all epithelia exhibit an exposed free surface and a basal surface which rests on a basement membrane and underlying vascularized connective tissue. This arrangement is requisite since all epithelia are intrinsically avascular and rely on nutrients diffusing upward across the basement membrane for their continued viability. Collectively, epithelia are the most functionally diverse of the four basic tissue types which contributes to their structural multiformity.

An epithelium covers the outside of the body (skin) providing protection against desiccation, microorganisms, radiant energy and chemicals. Many epithelia are secretory in function and widely dispersed where they produce sweat, tears, mucous, sebum, hydrochloric acid, digestive enzymes, hormones, bile salts, urine, milk, enamel matrix and reproductive cells. Others are important in provision of nutrients for all other cells of the body through their absorptive roles (intestinal epithelium) while specialized types use these raw substances for synthesis of energy-rich storage materials (liver and kidney cells). Some provide a barrier which allows selective passage of gases, fluids or metabolites (vascular endothelium, mesothelium of serosa, epithelium of the nephron, respiratory alveolar epithelium). Certain epithelial cells possess motile structures (cilia) allowing them to propel substances or cells within the luminal cavity which they border (conducting portion of respiratory tract, part of the female reproductive tract) while others aid in propulsion of secretory substances within epithelial-lined secretory units (myoepithelial cells of various glands). Highly specialized forms act as sensory receptors (transducers) providing information to the central nervous system for integration and appropriate responses.

Epithelia are equally diverse in their embryologic origin and epithelial representatives of all three primary germ layers (ectoderm, mesoderm and endoderm) persist postnatally. Each specific type of epithelium is derived from a single germ layer and it is worthwhile to have a generalized idea of their embryologic derivation. Most of the epithelium forming the skin and its adnexal structures including the mammary glands as well as that lining the oral cavity, nasal cavities, and anus is derived from ectoderm. At least one pair of the major salivary glands (parotid) and the enamel-forming epithelium of tooth germs (ameloblastic layer) are derived from ectoderm as well.
Epithelia originating from endoderm line the gastrointestinal and

respiratory tracts and contribute the functional cells of the liver and gallbladder, pancreas, adenohypophysis, parathyroids, submandibular and sublingual salivary glands, urinary bladder and vagina. Mesodermal derivatives include the outer layer of serous membranes (mesothelium) and the lining of the heart and all blood vessels (endothelium). Epithelia comprising the adrenal cortex, uterus, male and female sex glands, and the nephron and collecting system of the kidney, which includes the renal pelves and ureters, are mesodermal in origin.

## Classification of Epithelial Tissues

The traditional classification of epithelial tissues is one of convenience and typically three general subtypes are recognized. These include:

1) Surfacing epithelia

2) Secreting epithelia (glands)

3) Special epithelia

In reality, all epithelia are surfacing epithelia since by definition they line or cover a body surface, however, some types are highly specialized to function in secretion, sensory reception or gamete production and are justifiable segregated.

## Surfacing Epithelia

Surfacing epithelia are distinguished by two characteristics. These are:

1) Number of cell layers involved in their formation.
   a) Simple epithelia - one cell layer
   b) Stratified epithelia - two or more cell layers

2) Shape and height of individual cells comprising the epithelium.

   a) Squamous - flat
   b) Cuboidal - height approximately equal to width
   c) Columnar - height greater than width

In certain cases, the free apical surfaces of epithelial cells are modified for specialized function and these characteristics can be used to further subclassify the specific type of epithelium. In total, eight types of surfacing epithelia are recognized. Included are four types of simple epithelia and four types of stratified epithelia.

1) Simple surfacing epithelia

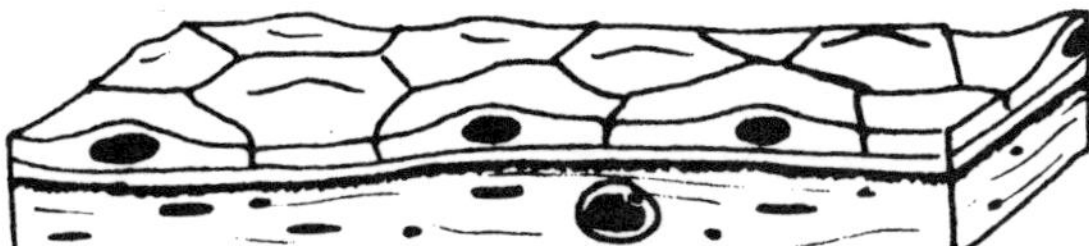
Simple Squamous Epithelium

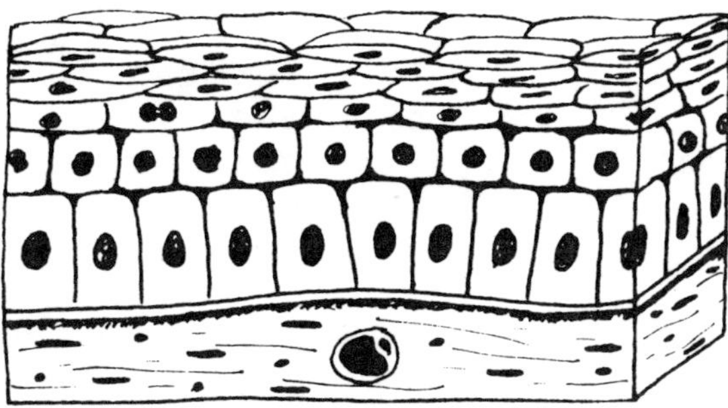
Stratified Squamous Epithelium (Moist)

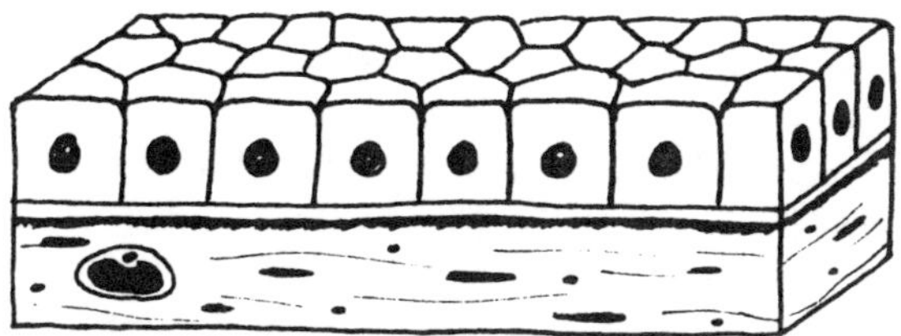
Simple Cuboidal Epithelium

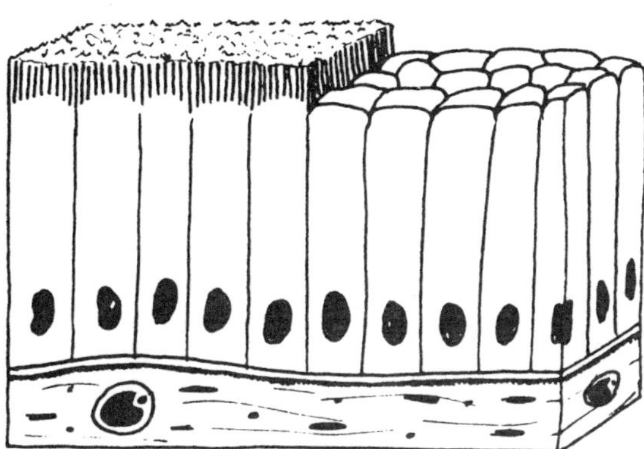
Simple Columnar Epithelium (Cilia on left)

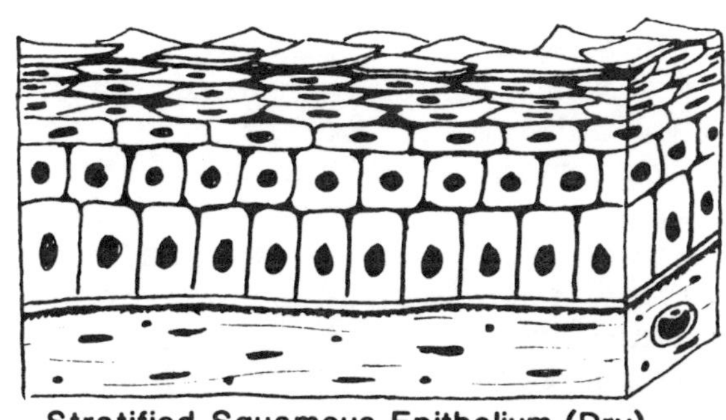
Stratified Squamous Epithelium (Dry)

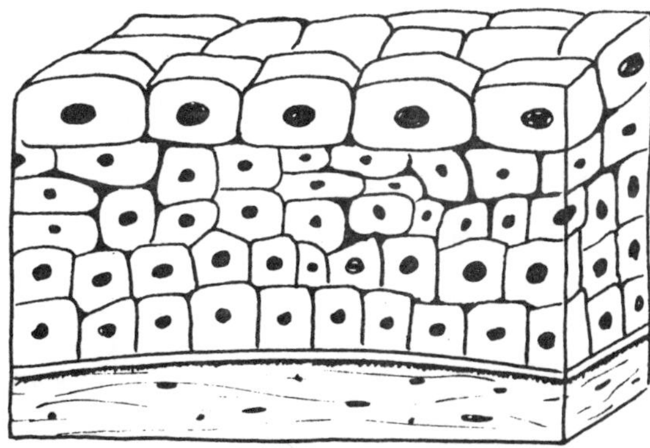
Transitional Epithelium (Urothelium)

**Fig. 2.1.** Major forms of epithelia

a) One layer of cells connected to underlying vascularized connective tissue by its basement membrane

b) The cell shape may be squamous, cuboidal or columnar

i) Simple squamous - extremely flattened, scale-like cells with the long axis of the nuclei lying parallel to the basement membrane. These cells are often so flat that the nucleus may cause the cell to bulge slightly because of its presence. Because of cytoplasmic thinness, this type of epithelium facilitates exchange of gases, metabolites or fluids. Locations include the lining of all blood and lymphatic vessels (endothelium), the serosal surfaces of viscera and lining of many closed body cavities (mesothelium), parietal layer of Bowman's capsule and the thin segment of the loop of Henle (both in the kidneys) and the alveoli of the lungs.

ii) Simple cuboidal - width and height nearly equal, surface view polyhedral, nuclei round to oval. This type of epithelium lines the ducts of many glands. Also found in proximal and distal convoluted tubules of the kidney, rete testis, germinal layer of ovary and secretory portions of some glands. Often exhibits border modifications including striated or brush borders and may be secretory or absorptive in function.

iii) Simple columnar - surface similar to cuboidal but height is greater than width, ovoid nuclei usually basally located with long axis oriented perpendicular to basement membrane. Primarily associated with secretion and absorption. Found in ducts of many glands and as a lining of: much of the gastrointestinal tract, small bronchi of lung, fallopian tube and uterus.

iv) Pseudostratified columnar - a special type of simple epithelium which appears to be stratified because not all cells reach the free surface so that they appear crowded and the nuclei stratify at different levels. It is regarded as a simple variety because all cells rest on the basement membrane. Cells are irregular in shape and height with the long axis of the nuclei perpendicular to the basement membrane.

Apical border modifications are usually present (cilia or stereocilia). Functionally, this epithelium plays a role in secretion and absorption and when cilia are present it is capable of moving intraluminal substances and cells across its free surface. This type of epithelium lines a large portion of the respiratory passages, the eustachian tube, part of the middle ear, ductus deferens and ductus epididymis. In the respiratory tract, the cells are often ciliated and unicellular glands (goblet cells) are present. When present in the male reproductive tract, the apical surface is usually covered with stereocilia, a variety of microvilli.

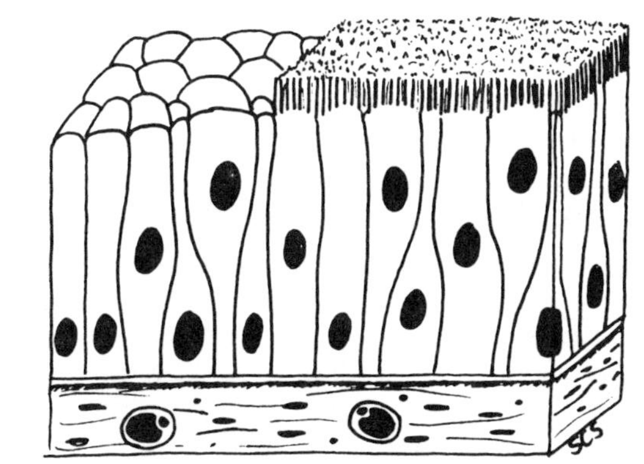

Pseudostratified columnar epithelium (Cilia on right)

**Fig. 2.2.** Pseudostratified columnar epithelium

2) Stratified surfacing epithelia
   a) Two or usually more cell layers are present.
   b) Only the basal layer of cells rests on the basement membrane.
   c) In most cases, the stratified epithelium is named according to the most superficial layer of cells which may be squamous, cuboidal or columnar. An additional type is referred to as transitional. As a group, the stratified epithelia are best suited to act as a protective barrier. They cover body surfaces most subject to wear, tear, stress or strain.
   d) There are four types of stratified epithelium.

      i) Stratified squamous epithelium - this type of epithelium is composed of many layers of cells of varying shape but it derives its name from its surface cells which are flattened and scale-like. Cells in subjacent layers may be columnar, cuboidal or polyhedral but become progressively flattened as they near the free surface. There are two variants of stratified squamous epithelium depending on whether the surface cells contain nuclei or cytoplasmic keratin.

1) Keratinized (cornified or dry) type - surface cells are flat and anucleate and are thus nonviable. The cytoplasm contains the protein, keratin, which is associated with tonofilaments. Tonofibrils and cell junctions are abundant. This type is adapted to resist abrasions and prevents desiccation and overhydration of underlying cells and tissues. It is found covering all of the outer surface of the body except the cornea. Portions of the oral cavity (gingiva, hard palate) which are normally nonkeratinized may become secondarily keratinized in man.

2) Nonkeratinized (moist or mucous) type - outermost layers are flat and contain dark (pycnotic) nuclei. Cells are still viable. Keratin is not normally formed, epithelial surface is moist. Underlying cells vary in shape and may be columnar, cuboidal or polygonal. Well-developed cellular junctions are present. Found as linings of moist cavities that open onto the body surface including the mouth, pharynx, esophagus and vagina.

ii) Stratified cuboidal epithelium - limited distribution, usually two cell layers present. Found lining the ducts of some glands.

iii) Stratified columnar epithelium - also limited in distribution. May be found at the interface of epithelial transition from one type to another where it serves to adjust for differences in epithelial thickness. Also lines some larger ducts of glands and is said to be present in part of the male urethra.

iv) Transitional epithelium (urothelium) - originally called "transitional" because it was believed to be a form intermediate between stratified squamous and stratified columnar. Urothelium is appropriate since it defines its location but is inadequate in describing its appearance. It is a stratified type in which the surface layer consists of dome-shaped cells. Surface cells are occasionally binucleate and often larger than the cells of underlying layers. Subjacent layers are co-lumnar, cuboidal or polyhedral in shape. It has unique flexible qualities and its morpho-logy varies with the degree of distention or contraction. Location is limited to the urinary tract where it is found lining the renal pelves, ureters, urinary bladder and the initial segment of the urethra.

## Epithelial membranes

An epithelium in combination with its underlying connective tissue constitutes a membrane. These vary in durability and thickness and of course in the type and arrangement of the cells of the epithelial component. Membranes are present as the mucosa of the gastrointestinal, respiratory and genitourinary systems. In these, the connective tissue is fine but closely woven resulting in a membrane that is capable of stretching but in which sufficient strength is present to prevent separation of the epithelial cells. In the skin, the underlying connective tissue is coarser and more fibrous, an arrangement which is suited to meet the requirements of a membrane that is subjected to frequent physical stress. There are two specific types of membranes. Classification as one or the other depends on their location and composition.

1) Serous membranes - line closed cavities and do not contain glands (the epithelium is not a secreting epithelium). They consist of a mesothelium and a subjacent layer of delicate fibroelastic connective tissue. Serous membranes are found as linings of the peritoneal, pleural and pericardial cavities. They are moistened by a thin fluid that is compositionally similar to lymph.

2) Mucous membranes - line the cavities and tubular organs that communicate with the exterior. They consist of a surfacing epithelium, its underlying basement membrane and subjacent connective tissue termed the lamina propria. Glands may be present but are not required for inclusion in this category. The glands, when present, may be mucous as the name implies but serous glands may be found as well. Mucous membranes line the alimentary tracts and major respiratory passages in which both mucous and serous glands may be integrated. They also are present as the linings of portions of the genitourinary tract where they are usually not

associated with glands.

## Secreting Epithelia

Secreting epithelia are surfacing epithelia that retain the basic features of such but are specialized particularly for the role of secretion. More commonly they are referred to as glandular epithelia or simply glands and when they are the major component of an organ, it may be referred to as a gland. As a generalization, the cells of secretory epithelia are found in a single layer (simple). One exception to this is sebaceous glands in which the cells are present in a stratified arrangement. Another conceptual generalization that can be made about glands is that they are developmentally derived from general surfacing epithelia beneath which in certain instances they proliferate to become discrete structures connected to the surface by a duct. The duct may be quite simple or extremely complex with functions of its own or in specific cases the duct may subsequently degenerate. In the latter instance, the glands must use an alternate pathway to disseminate their secretory products.

Glands may be single cells or groups of cells. They may be part of the surface layer or may reside below connected to it through a ductal system or when their communication to the surface is developmentally sacrificed, they may secrete directly into the vascular system. For the most part, glandular epithelial cells do not possess surface modifications because they are not required for secretory function. In many cases, the intracellular components of a cell indicate its secretory nature and the type of secretory product.

The classification of glands can be made extremely complex but in a practical sense such an approach is not necessary for an understanding of their function or an appreciation of their structural diversity. Glands which release their secretory product into a duct are referred to as exocrine glands while those which ultimately use the vascular system are referred to as endocrine glands. Some of the endocrine glands are not epithelial derivatives and in those cases the generalizations concerning epithelially-derived glands may not apply. The endocrine glands will be studied in a subsequent section on the endocrine system. The exocrine glands can be classified on the basis of four characteristics:

1) Number of component cells (unicellular or multicellular).
2) Complexity of the ductal system (simple or compound) and the structure of the secretory component (tubular or alveolar or tubuloalveolar).
3) Type of secretory product (serous or mucous or seromucous).
4) Mode of secretion (merocrine or apocrine or holocrine).

## Unicellular Glands

A unicellular gland represents the simplest glandular structure. It consists of a single secretory cell interposed between nonsecretory cells of the general surfacing epithelium. The most appropriate example of this type is the mucous-producing goblet cell, a resident cell of certain parts of the respiratory and gastrointestinal tracts. By light microscopy the goblet cell is characterized by the presence of abundant, lightly-stained supranuclear secretory granules and a nucleus that is located basally and flattened. When the goblet cell is present as an isolated unit, the accumulation of mucous within the apical cytoplasm tends to cause bulging of the lateral cell borders into the domain of adjacent cells devoid of mucous. A combination of the above features results in the characteristic flask-like shape of the goblet cell.

## Multicellular Glands

Various forms belong to this category but two main types bear further consideration. They are:

1) Mucous secreting sheet - in this form, the mucous secreting cells (unicellular glands) have become so concentrated that they represent a glandular surfacing epithelium. Since nearly all the cells are secretory, an essential element necessary to produce the appearance of the goblet cell (secretory cells mixed with nonsecretory cells) is not present. The mucous-secreting sheet represents the final developmental step in which the general surfacing epithelium is still capable of meeting its secretory requirements. Additional secretory demands necessitate the development of subsurface glands, connected to the surface by ducts. Such an arrangement serves to increase the secretory surface without increasing the usually fixed dimensions of the structure in which the glands are located. The cells of the mucous secreting sheet are separated from each other by regularly parallel lateral borders, contain oval, lightly stained nuclei and an apical cytoplasm in which a cup-like mass of mucous may be found.

2) True glands - in these, the term exocrine is applied since the secretory component lies below the general surfacing epithelium and is connected to it by a duct through which the secretory product passes. Depending upon the complexity of the ductal system, the glands are be said to be simple if the duct remains unbranched or compound if branching occurs. The simple and compound glands can be further subclassified by the complexity of the secretory portion. This latter

feature is difficult to access in a single tissue section in which only two dimensions are represented but the concept is important from a didactic standpoint. Features and sample locations of the more common configurations of glands follows:

a) Simple tubular glands - these are the simplest of the true glands and represent the earliest developmental stage in which divergence of glandular surfacing epithelia and true subsurface glands occurs.

   i) Straight simple tubular glands - single unbranched tubular duct with single tubular secretory unit. Example: crypts of Lieberkuhn in the small intestine.
   ii) Coiled simple tubular glands - unbranched duct and secretory unit both tubular, secretory unit convoluted. Example: eccrine sweat glands in dermis of skin.
   iii) Simple branched tubular glands - duct single and unbranched, secretory units are branched and tubular in shape. Example: Brunner's glands in the duodenum.
   iv) Simple branched alveolar (acinar) glands - duct single and unbranched, secretory units branched and sac-like. Example: sebaceous glands (Note: sebaceous glands are unusual in that the cells lining the alveoli (acini) are stratified and secrete by the holocrine mode).

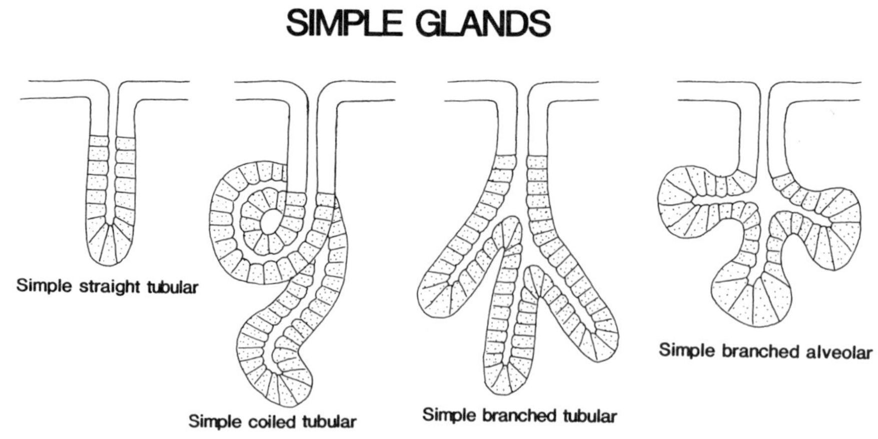

**Fig. 2.3.** Types of simple glands

b) Compound glands - characterized by branching of the duct so that a ductal system with increasing smaller diameters is present. The secretory units are also multiple and may be all tubular or a mixture of tubular and alveolar.

i) Compound tubular glands - branched ductal system, branched tubular secretory units. Example: glands in cardia of stomach.

ii) Compound tubuloalveolar glands - branched ductal system, some secretory units tubular others sac-like (alveolar or acinar). Example: Pancreas, salivary glands.

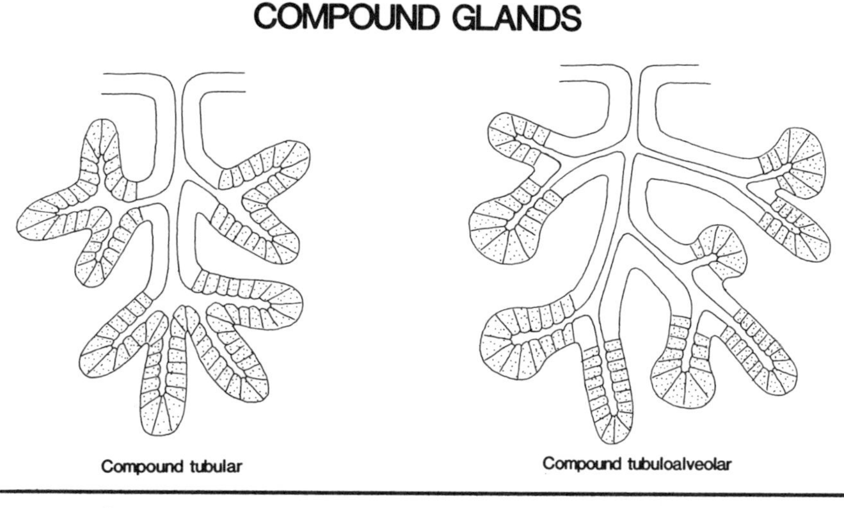


**Fig. 2.4.** Types of compound glands

## Nature and Mode of Secretion

Glands can also be classified based on the nature of the secretory material produced by the secretory units and by the mode in which they secrete it.

1) The glandular secretion may be serous, mucous or seromucous (mixed).
   a) Serous glands - secrete a clear, watery fluid containing protein. The nuclei of the glandular acinar cells are round and lightly-stained and the lumen of the acinus is imperceptible. Example: parotid salivary gland is purely serous.
   b) Mucous glands - secrete mucous which is a viscous substance composed primarily of a glycoprotein, mucin, plus water. The cells of the acini stain lightly and possess a dark-stained, basally-located flattened nucleus. The acinar lumen is usually visualized. Example: Brunner's glands of duodenum are purely mucous.

c) <u>Seromucous glands</u> - also referred to as mixed glands, these have both a serous and a mucous component. Each may occupy different acini (serous units and mucous units) or they may share the same acinus as a mucous unit covered externally by a crescent of serous cells (serous demilune). Example: submandibular salivary gland is seromucous.

## GLANDULAR UNITS

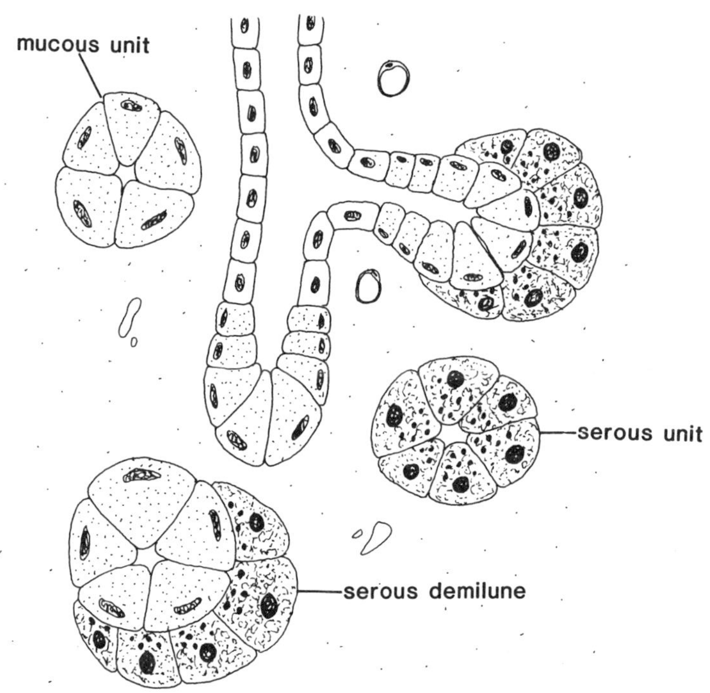


**Fig. 2.5.** Serous, mucous and seromucous units

2) The mode of secretion may be merocrine (eccrine), apocrine or holocrine.
   a) <u>Merocrine</u> - discharge of membrane-bound secretory granule by fusion with plasma membrane without disrupting it. Examples: Pancreas and salivary glands.
   b) <u>Apocrine</u> - apical surface of cell and enclosed secretory product "buds off" with resultant loss of some of the apical plasma membrane and cytoplasm. Examples: Apocrine sweat glands and mammary gland.
   c) <u>Holocrine</u> - in this type the entire cell is lost into the duct along with its contained secretory product. Example: Sebaceous glands.

### Special Epithelia

To this category belong such diverse epithelia as those involved in special sensory perception, in production of male germ cells (spermatocytes) or tooth enamel as well as ones specialized for filtration of the blood (kidney podocytes). These will be discussed more fully in appropriate sections.

## CONNECTIVE TISSUE

Like epithelial tissue, connective tissue is remarkably heterogeneous and includes a diversity of specialized structures ranging from osseous and cartilaginous tissue to seemingly unrelated entities such as blood, bone marrow and lymphoid tissue. Other structures with more generalized properties such as tendons, ligaments, fasciae and subepithelial connective tissue belong in the category of connective tissue as well and are often collectively referred to as the connective tissues proper. As a group, the connective tissues play an important role in the provision and maintenance of body form, hence, their name. Unlike the other three basic tissues (epithelial, muscle and nervous), in which cells are the chief constituent, connective tissue is composed mainly of extracellular material produced largely by its sparse cell population. The fundamental cell primarily responsible for manufacture and secretion of the extracellular material (matrix) is the fibroblast, a derivative of embryonal mesenchyme. The matrix is responsible for the supportive characteristics and depending upon the specific type of connective tissue in which it is found, is composed of various fibers and an amorphous, viscous fluid known as ground substance. The classification of the connective tissues is based either on the characteristic of the cell population or on the characteristics of the components of the extracellular matrix (fibers or ground substance).

### Embryonal Connective Tissue

There are two subtypes within this category. The first, mesenchyme, has generalized properties while the second, mucous connective tissue possesses properties that are more specialized.

#### Mesenchyme

Mesenchyme is derived from embryonic mesoderm and is the first connective tissue to develop in the embryo. It is the most undifferentiated type and is the precursor for the subsequent development of all other types of connective tissue. It is characterized by sparse numbers of stellate-shaped cells embedded in abundant amorphous intercellular matrix. The main feature which differentiates this form from all other types of connective tissue is the absence of fibers in the matrix. Normally, at birth, little mesenchyme is present since most of the mesenchymal cell have differentiated into functional fibroblasts or other types of mesenchymally-derived cells (muscle cells, endothelial cells, mesothelial cells, fat cells, chrondroblasts, osteoblasts, reticulum cells and the parenchymal cells of some glands). In the adult, mesenchyme is restricted to the pregnant uterus where it contributes to the embryonic and fetal membranes.

### Mucous Connective Tissue

This type is a special embryonic and fetal connective tissue that bears resemblance to mesenchyme but in addition to those common features its matrix contains a minor component of very small fibers and its ground substance has a gelatinous consistency. Because of the latter characteristic, it is often referred to as "Wharton's jelly". In the embryo, fetus and newborn it is restricted almost entirely to the umbilical cord. In the adult, the vitreous body of the eye and the pulp of young teeth are considered by some to be types of mucous connective tissue.

## Adult Connective Tissue

The adult connective tissues are the ones most usually encountered in the study of tissues. They can be subclassified by the nature of their function. Those whose functions are more generalized are amalgamated into a category known as the connective tissue proper while those whose functions are more specialized (cartilaginous, osseous and reticular connective tissues) are segregated by the nature of their extracellular matrices (ground substance and fibers) and specific cell populations which are intimately related to the performance of their histophysiologic tasks.

### Connective Tissue Cells

The functional cell of the connective tissue proper is the fibroblast. It synthesizes the fibers and the ground substances. When actively synthesizing, the fibroblast is characterized by an abundant, irregularly branched cytoplasm which is difficult to visualize in routine preparations at the light microscopic level. Its nucleus is ovoid, vesicular and contains a prominent nucleolus. In electron micrographs, the fibroblast contains cytoplasmic and nuclear organelles associated with protein synthesis (abundant RER, prominent Golgi and active-appearing nucleoli). When the fibroblast is quiescent (not synthesizing), it is spindle-shaped with a dark, elongated nucleus and when in this functional and morphologic state it is sometimes referred to as a fibrocyte. The cells of the connective tissue proper can be organized into two categories:

1) Stable or nonmigratory cell population

2) Migratory cell population

The first category may contain, besides the fibroblast or fibrocyte, various numbers of mast cells, fat cells and plasma cells. The migratory cell population is highly variable in terms of cell types and quantities of each and includes macrophages, tissue neutrophils, tissue eosinophils and lymphocytes. All of the cells in the migratory population as well as the mast cells and plasma cells of the stable population are involved in inflammatory and immune-related responses in which the connective tissues play and important but often underestimated role.

The adult connective tissues with specialized functions contain cells that are specifically adapted to their functional roles. The functional cell of osseous tissue is the osteoblast. It synthesizes a specialized matrix known as osteoid composed predominately of collagen fibers which, with the addition of inorganic salts, becomes secondarily mineralized into a hard tissue. Cartilagineous tissue contains various types of fibers and a functional cell type (chondroblast) which secretes a specialized ground substance. The predominate structural component of reticular connective tissue is its functional cell, the reticulum cell, although fibers (reticular) and ground substance is present as well. It should be noted that all three of the specialized adult connective tissues contain the basic elements of connective tissues (cells, fibers and ground substance) but that in each a different one assumes chief functional importance.

## Connective Tissue Fibers

There are three types of fibers that occur in the connective tissues: collagen, elastic and reticular. Fiber density, arrangement and quantity relates to the functional requirements of the particular type of connective tissue.

1) Collagen fibers - present to some degree in all connective tissues. Collagen a polymer of monomeric (tropocollagen) units. Fibroblasts, chrondroblasts and osteoblasts produce and secrete monomeric tropocollagen which subsequently polymerizes extracellularly. Because of the geometric arrangement of the polymerized tropocollagen molecules, collagen is characterized by 64 nm periodicity observable at the ultrastructural level. Epithelial cells are thought to produce a peculiar type of collagen lacking periodicity which is deposited in their basal lamina. The tropocollagen molecule is composed of three polypeptide chains (alpha units) which are rich in glycine and proline and contains two amino acids, hydroxyproline and hydroxylysine, not usually found in other proteins. The alpha units (chains) consist of three amino acids.

The initial amino acid can be any amino acid except proline or lysine. The second is always proline or lysine while the third is always glycine. As indicated above the lysine or proline molecules may be hydroxylated. Hydroxylysine is responsible for crosslinking between collagen fibers which contributes to their tensile strength. Vitamin C is an important cofactor required for the enzymatic conversion of proline to hydroxyproline. Therefore, a deficiency of vitamin C may result in faulty collagen biosynthesis, a condition known clinically as scurvy. There are five types of collagen based on the type and arrangement of the alpha units:

a) Type I - most abundant, widespread distribution, 64 nm periodicity. Easily visualized especially if present in bundles. Locations: dermis, bone, tendon, dentin, organ capsules, fasciae, sclera, fibrocartilage.
b) Type II - present mainly in cartilage (hyaline and elastic), not readily visible with routine techniques. 64 nm periodicity. Location: hyaline and elastic cartilage.
c) Type III - argyrophilic and PAS+, not visualized with routine stains. Very thin collagen fibers produced by reticulum cells (reticular fibers). Same periodicity as Type I. Location: reticular connective tissue.
d) Type IV - produced by some epithelial and endothelial cells. Lacks periodicity. Location: basal laminae.
e) Type V - poorly characterized. Lacks periodicity. Location: placental basal lamina.

2) <u>Reticular fibers</u> - actually very thin collagen fibers, not arranged into bundles, best visualized by silver stains (argyrophilic) and because of their carbohydrate moieties they are PAS positive. They contribute a delicate supporting network to many tissues and organs and constitute the framework for hematopoietic and lymphoid tissues and organs.

3) <u>Elastic fibers</u> - composed of an amorphous protein termed elastin, are quite thin and lack periodicity. They are not visualized unless special staining techniques are employed. Like collagen, elastin is rich in glycine and proline but in addition it contains two uncommon amino acids, desmosine and isodesmosine and is rich in valine as well. Elastic fibers are found wherever flexibility is required including the walls of certain arteries, trachea, trabeculae of the spleen, ligamentum flava and skin. They are, of course, present as part of the fiber population of

elastic cartilage along with Type II collagen fibers.

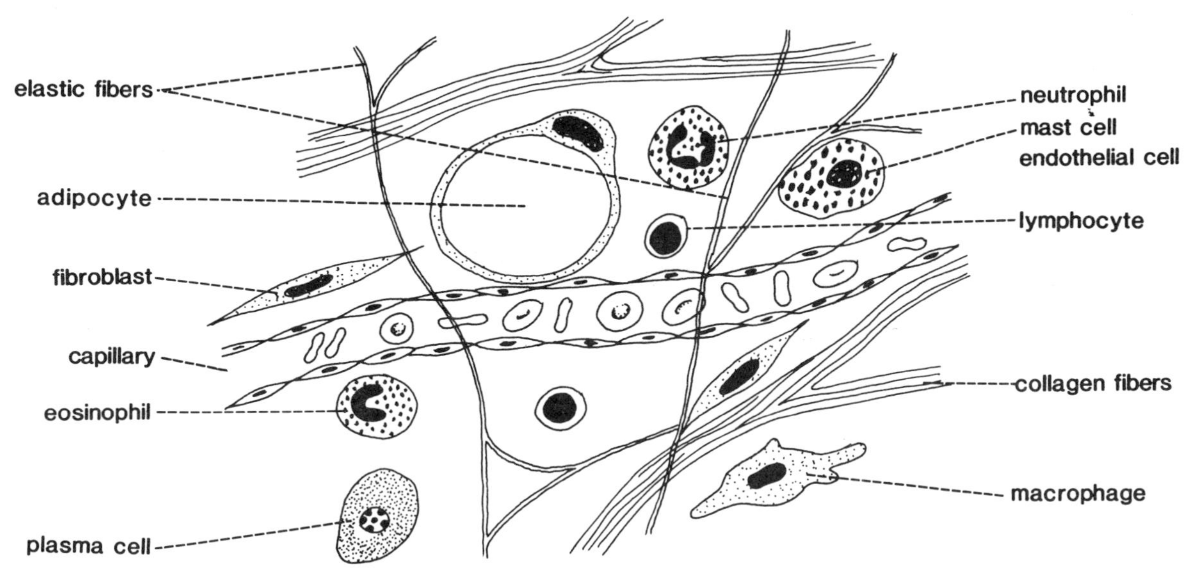


**Fig. 2.6.** Types of cells and fibers of connective tissue

## Ground Substance

The ground substance of connective tissues is a colorless, transparent and homogeneous colloidal substance which constitutes both a molecular sieve and a physical barrier to the spread of larger molecules. It is adept at binding water and serves as a medium for the bidirectional diffusion of gases and metabolic materials between blood vessels and the connective tissues cells embedded within it. Besides water and ions, the ground substance of the connective tissue proper contains structural glycoproteins and glycosaminoglycans (GAGs) which contribute to its viscosity and other properties. GAGs are linear polysaccharide molecules of repeating disaccharide units composed of a particular hexosamine and a uronic acid. The acid may be either glucuronate or iduronate while the hexosamine may be either glucosamine or galactosamine. Hyaluronate is the major component of the ground substance of the connective tissue proper.

With the exception of hyaluronate, the GAGs are covalently bound to a protein core to form larger molecules known as proteoglycans. Hyaluronate is the only nonsulfated GAG, and thus is not normally demonstrated in routine tissue sections. The sulfated proteoglycans, dermatan sulfate, chondroitin sulfate, keratan and heparan sulfate bear a net negative charge and stain with basic dyes and to a lesser extent with hematoxylin. The sulfated proteoglycans have a wide distribution in connective tissues and are present in appreciable quantities in cartilages and the cornea.

## Connective Tissue Proper

This group is the least specialized of the adult connective tissues. The three most commonly recognized subtypes are:

1) Loose Irregular (Areolar) Connective Tissue- this is the prototype of the connective tissue proper and consists of the basic three components: cells, fibers and ground substance. The cell population is sparse and extremely heterogeneous. Representatives of any or all of the stable and migratory populations may be present. The functional cell in this category, as well as in the next two, is the fibroblast which produces the fibers (mostly Type I collagen) and the ground substance (mostly hyaluronic acid). It is characterized by its loose nature and by nearly equal proportions of fibers and ground substance. Locations: found in association with many types of epithelia and vascular structures.

2) Dense Irregular Connective Tissue - the basic structure bears similarities to that of areolar connective tissue but differs in that the collagen fibers are greater in number and present in bundles which are easily visualized. Consequently as the quantity of collagen fibers increases per unit area the amount of space left to be filled by the ground substance decreases. In dense irregular connective tissue, thick collagen bundles are present in a random, haphazard arrangement, a feature which is reflected by its descriptive appellation. Any of the cell types found in areolar connective tissue may be present. Normally, the vast majority of cells are fibroblasts (and/or fibrocytes) which secrete the collagen fibers (mostly Type I) and ground substance. Locations: an excellent example is the dermis of the skin but other sites include capsules of some organs and the outer investments of nerves.

3) Dense Regular Connective Tissue - in this type the collagen bundles are regularly arranged and occupy most of the space so that little room is left to be filled by ground substance. As a result the cell population is quite small and almost all the cells (greater than 95%) are fibroblasts (and/or fibrocytes). The fibroblasts are elongated to conform to the minimal space left by the regular packed collagen fibers. Locations: tendons and ligaments.

The segregation of the above subtypes is based largely on the quantity and arrangement of their matrix fibers, all of which consist of the protein, collagen. The functional cell type in all three is the fibroblast. In addition to these three subtypes, other types containing an abundance of a certain cell or fiber type receive alternate designations. These include:

1) Adipose connective tissue - also termed adipose tissue, it represents areolar connective tissue in which large numbers of fat cells (adipocytes) are present. Unlike other types of connective tissue proper, it is the cell population (fat cells) and not the extracellular matrix that makes up the bulk of the tissue. Example: subcutaneous connective tissue is adipose connective tissue.
2) Fibrofatty connective tissue - whereas fatty connective tissue represents areolar connective tissue in which fat cells are found in such abundance that they are its major component, fibrofatty connective tissue is simply dense irregular connective tissue in which large numbers of fat cells are aggregated. It is a transitional form of connective tissue found at the interface of the usual variety of dense irregular connective tissue (such as that present in the dermis of the skin) and the underlying adipose connective tissue of the subcutis.

3) Pigmented connective tissue - this connective tissue variant contains large numbers of melanin pigment-containing cells termed melanophores. It is found within the choroid layer and iris of the eye.

4) Elastic connective tissue - although small numbers of elastic fibers may be present in almost all connective tissues and are especially prominent in the elastic type of cartilaginous tissue to be discussed subsequently, in some areas the elastic fibers predominate in number over collagen or reticular fibers. In this case, the special designation, elastic connective tissue, is sometimes used. This variant is found in various anatomic structures including the ligamenta flava between the vertebrae, anterior abdominal wall fasciae, trachea and bronchi, vocal cords, walls of the aorta and other elastic arteries and suspensory ligament of the penis.

## Special Connective Tissue

There are three types of connective tissue with specialized properties. These include cartilaginous tissue, osseous tissue and reticular connective tissue. The three entities included in this category are highly specialized in form and function but are still composed of the three basic elements common to all connective tissues: cells, fibers and ground substance.

The above terms are used to describe the special connective tissues when they are studied at a level which largely ignores any interaction with other types of tissue. For example, osseous tissue and bone denote different levels of structural complexity and functional specialization. Osseous tissue is a specialized form of connective tissue which contains cells (osteoblasts) that synthesize and secrete bone matrix (osteoid) composed chiefly of Type I collagen fibers. The osteoid is subsequently mineralized to form the hard tissue component of what is recognized grossly as a bone (For example: the femur). Careful study of a growing long bone reveals that it is a complex arrangement of various tissues (an organ) which interact to achieve functional specialization. The contribution of osseous tissue is apparent but other types of connective tissues may be found that not only contribute to its structural complexities but are related to its diverse functions as well. Cartilaginous tissue (hyaline type) in the form of an epiphyseal plate is present which is converted to osseous tissue to effect growth in length. Bone marrow (a type of reticular connective tissue involved in hematopoiesis) may be found in the medullary cavity. Dense regular or irregular connective tissue forms part of the periosteal covering of the bone. The other three basic tissues may be represented as well. Blood vessels, lined by endothelium (an epithelial tissue) and at certain levels surrounded by layers of smooth muscle cells (muscular tissue), are an integral component of a bone. In fact, the presence of vascular elements and their proximity to the osteogenic cells is paramount in bone histogenesis, reflected ultimately by its microscopic arrangement. Both myelinated and unmyelinated nerves (nervous tissue) are present within the periosteum. They follow the vessels as they enter the bone. Both efferent (vascular smooth muscle contraction) and afferent (periosteal pain) modalities are represented.

It is obvious that the synonymous use of the term "bone" to describe a single tissue component (osseous tissue) of the complex organ in which it is found as well as the organ itself leads to confusion in the conceptual distinction between tissue and organ. The reader should be aware of the semantical problems which imprecision of terminology can create and that the terminology used here, although correct, is not universal by any means.

## Cartilaginous Tissue

The same semantic difficulties described above are also encountered in the use of the term "cartilage" which is at times used to describe discrete cartilaginous structures (such as a tracheal or laryngeal cartilage) consisting of cartilaginous tissue admixed and interacting with other types of tissue (a cartilaginous organ) while in other instances it is used interchangeably with cartilaginous tissue (such as that found in an epiphyseal plate) present as a component of a more complex structure (in this example an organ, the growing long bone).

Cartilaginous tissue is a specialized, semirigid tissue subdivided into three morphologic types: hyaline, elastic and fibrous. All three types can be described by their components: cells, fibers and ground substance. The last two components (fibers and ground substance) are collectively termed the extracellular matrix which differs in each type providing the basis for their morphologic and biochemical distinction. The ground substance is the specialized component of cartilaginous tissue.

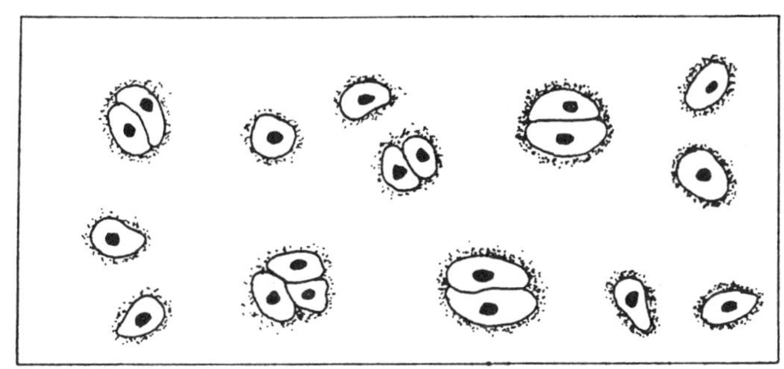

Hyaline cartilage

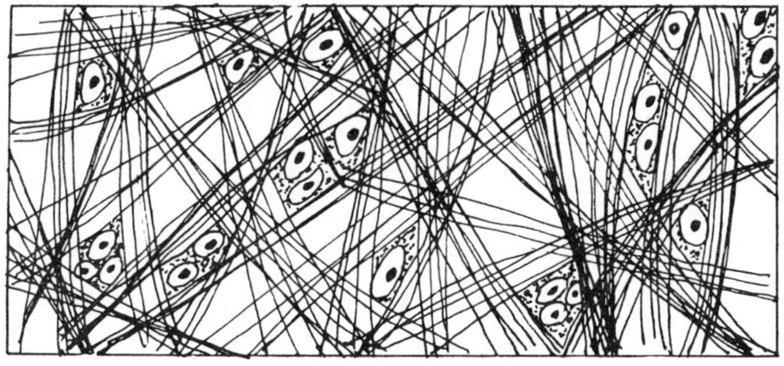

Elastic cartilage

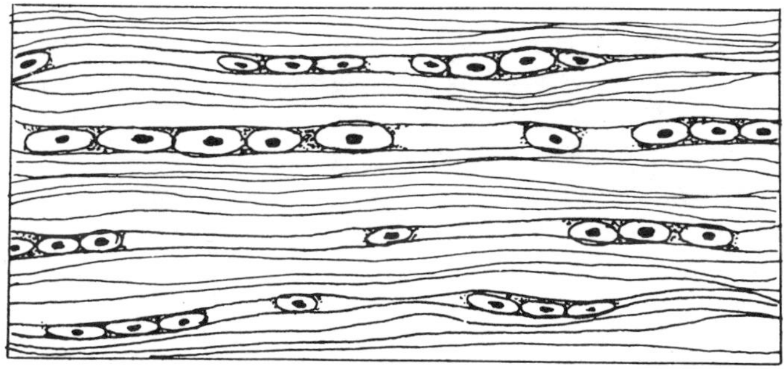

Fibrocartilage

**Fig. 2.7.** Three types of cartilaginous tissue. (Courtesy Dr. R. Snell)

The functional cells of all three subtypes are referred to as chondroblasts until they secrete enough extracellular matrix so that they are completely surrounded by it, at which time, they are called chondrocytes. Both chondroblasts and chondrocytes possess the potential to secrete the components of the extracellular matrix.

1) Hyaline - located in the walls of the major respiratory passages (trachea and bronchi) as discrete cartilaginous organs. It functions elsewhere as costal, articular, nasal and epiphyseal growth plate connective tissue. Ground substance consists primarily of proteoglycans. These consist of a core of protein to which glycosaminoglycans (GAGs) are covalently linked. Most of the GAGs contain acidic sulfate moieties and are referred to as chondroitin sulfates. Due to the high concentration of polyanionic GAGs, the matrix has a high content of water (approximately 75%). This level of water allows nutrients to reach the chondrocytes by diffusion, a necessary arrangement since mature cartilaginous tissue is avascular. It also lends resiliency creating a shock absorber effect, a property which makes its suited to cover the surfaces of articulating bones. The fibrous component is Type II collagen. The fibers are not visible because they have the same refractive index as the ground substance resulting in a homogeneous, glassy appearance.

2) Elastic - typically found in the external ear, eustachian tube, epiglottis and the corniculate and cuneiform cartilages of the larynx. The ground substance is similar to that present in the hyaline type. Fibers consist of a mixture of Type II collagen fibers and elastic fibers. The elastic fibers are visible giving the matrix a heterogeneous appearance.

3) Fibrous - commonly found in regions requiring firm support, tensile strength and resistance to shearing forces. Such locations include intervertebral disks, pubic symphysis, certain joints and sites of tendinous and ligamentous attachments. Besides the chondrocytes, flattened fibroblasts are present in this type as well. Ground substance is similar to that produced by less specialized connective tissues and is largely hyaluronic acid present in small amounts. The fibers are composed of Type I collagen which are the major component of this type. Fibers are easily seen and in most examples are arrangely in parallel rows. Those of the vertebral discs present a more randomized, herringbone pattern. NOTE: Some authorities do not regard this as a specific subtype but rather dense fibrous connective tissues containing cartilage cells

or dense fibrous connective tissue mixed with a small amount of the hyaline type of cartilaginous tissue.

Growth occurs potentially by two mechanisms: appositional and interstitial. If a complete or partial external fibro-vascular investment (perichondrium) of the cartilaginous mass is present then appositional growth may occur at the interface of the perichondrium with the cartilaginous tissue. Mesenchymal cells in the perichondrium (chondrogenic layer) differentiate into chondroblasts which secrete extracellular matrix until they become chondrocytes entrapped in their own secretory product. This effectively adds cells and matrix to the outside.

Interstitial growth occurs when entrapped chondrocytes divide and begin to synthesize and secrete additional extracellular matrix. This effectively adds cells and matrix to the inside. Groups of newly divided cells are referred to as cell nests or isogenous groups. Recently secreted extracellular matrix in the vicinity of isogenous cell groups stains more basophilic and is called the territorial matrix. The older matrix is termed the interterritorial matrix and has a less basophilic appearance due in part to the dilutional effect of increased water binding of the extracellular matrix in this area.

## Osseous Tissue

Like other connective tissues, osseous tissue consists of cells, fibers and ground substance. The fibers are the specialized component of osseous tissue.

1) Cells - in developing and mature osseous tissue, four type of cells can be recognized:
   a) Osteoblasts are osteogenic cells which are capable of synthesis and secretion of the organic matrix (osteoid). They are characterized morphologically by a singular nucleus and by their peripheral position along mineralized surfaces. They may be found in a single layer lining the internal surfaces (endosteal layer) and as a specific component of the periosteum (osteogenic layer) of a mature bone. They contain the intracellular organelles of a typical protein-secreting cell and play an indirect role in mineralization of osteoid. Active osteoblasts contain an abundance of the enzyme, alkaline phosphatase, and like other protein synthesizing cells, they stain basophilic.
   b) Osteocytes are found in lacunae surrounded by the extracellular matrix that they secreted as an osteoblast. They form a canalicular system (cell-to-cell contacts, gap junctions) with other osteocytes and with osteoblasts. They are incapable of secreting extracellular matrix

because of their incarceration in hard tissue.

c) Osteoclasts are large multinucleated cells formed by the fusion of preosteoclasts which have a hematopoietic (monocytic) origin. They are often found within depressions (Howship's lacunae) on the surface of mineralized osseous tissue where they are active in resorption processes. When stained with hematoxylin and eosin, their cytoplasm appears eosinophilic. Ultrastructurally, they contain a paucity of granular endoplasmic reticulum but clusters of free ribosomes may be present. The cell surface opposed to the mineralized surface is characterized by the presence of numerous cytoplasmic processes and microvilli, the so-called "ruffled border". Lysosomes are particularly abundant and reflecting their multinuclear state, numerous paired centrioles and Golgi complexes may be identified. When active they contain an abundance of acid phosphatase corresponding to their lysosomal content.

d) Osteoprogenitor cells maintain the functional cell population by proliferation and differentiation into osteogenic cells (osteoblasts).

2) Extracellular matrix - as in other connective tissues, the extracellular matrix contains fibers and ground substance but, peculiar to osseous tissue, the matrix is secondarily impregnated with inorganic salts resulting in hardness and strength not present in other connective tissues. Thus, osseous tissue is suited to provide bone organs with their special properties. The extracellular matrix consists of an organic matrix (24%) and inorganic mineral (76%).

a) Organic matrix (osteoid) is composed of a fibrous component (90%) consisting of Type I collagen fibers and ground substance (10%) which is largely nonsulphated proteoglycans, but some keratan sulfate and chondroitin-4-sulfate are present in small quantities.

b) Inorganic material consists of crystals of calcium and phosphate in the form of hydroxyapatite, $[Ca_{10}(PO_4)_6OH_2]$.

## Organization of Skeletal Elements

The skeleton plays vital roles in physical support, protection of underlying organs and viscera, hematopoiesis and various homeostatic mechanisms including the provision of an immense calcium reservoir. It is appropriate and perhaps conceptually helpful to subdivide the skeletal elements by their functional level of organization. In descending order of complexity these include:

1) Skeletal level - this includes the boney skeleton as a whole.

2) Organ level - at this level, individual boney organs are recognized (For example: the tibia).

3) Complex tissue level - this level includes categories which possess differences that are probably the final ones still observable with the naked eye. These two categories and their differences are:
   a) Cortical (compact) organization of osseous tissue which is found on the outside (cortex) of many bones, especially the long bones. It is well-vascularized to provide metabolic support to the osteocytes which are embedded within it.
   b) Trabecular organization of osseous tissue. Also termed cancellous or spongy, this pattern is associated with the medullary cavities. Because of the thinness of the trabeculae and their proximity to the well-vascularized medullary cavity, the trabecular osseous tissue is poorly-vascularized.

4) Simple tissue level - it is at this level that microscopic differences are important. The two categories included here vary in the arrangement of the collagen fibers within the extracellular matrix.
   a) Woven - this pattern is characterized by a random arrangement of the collagen fibers. Considered an immature state, it is found in areas of rapid growth such as in the early developmental phases of both membranous and endochondral growth and associated with healing of fractures. It is eventually converted to a lamellar pattern.
   b) Lamellar - a highly ordered arrangement of the collagen fibers is present which lends to increased strength. This is the most important and frequent histoarchitectural pattern present in bone organs and is one the associated with the functional, repeating unit of bone organs, the osteon.

## The Osteon

The primary structural unit of compact osseous tissue is called the osteon or haversian system. It consists of lamellae (haversian lamellae) arranged in a concentric pattern around a central canal (haversian canal) that contains a blood vessel, nerves and a minor connective tissue component. Osteoprogenitor cells line the canal and osteocytes within lacunae are arranged concentrically about the canal toward which their canaliculi radiate. The osteons within the cortex of long bones are arranged parallel to the long axis of the bone. In some areas, the haversian canals anastomose freely with each other, while in others, vascular channels (Volkmann's canals) running roughly perpendicular to the long axis of haversian canals connect the haversian vessels of neighboring haversian systems or alternately they link the them with the external bone surface or the medullary cavity. The two canals can be distinguished not only by their differing spatial orientation but also by the fact that the Volkmann's canals, unlike the haversian canals, are not surrounded by concentric lamellae of osseous tissue. Like haversian systems, they contain a layer of osteoprogenitor cells. Besides the lamellae that surround the osteon, two other forms are present within bone organs.

SEGMENT OF HAVERSIAN SYSTEM

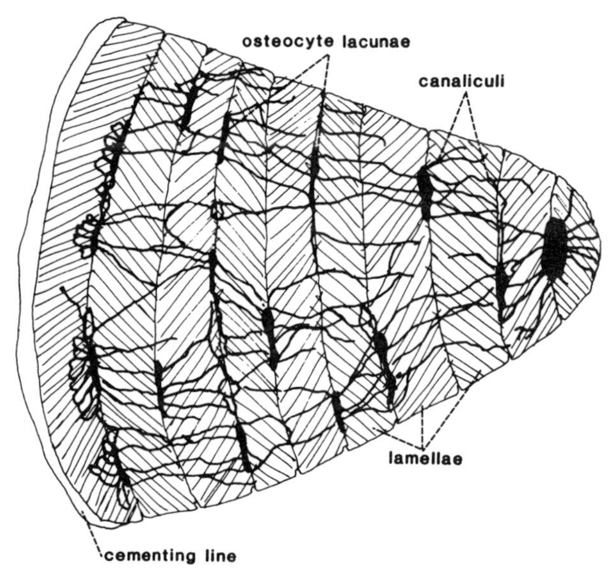


**Fig. 2.8.** Osteonal structure

1) Interstitial lamellae - these represent remnants of laminated osseous tissue left from older, partially resorbed and remodeled haversian systems that fill the irregularly-shaped areas not occupied by the roughly cylindrically-shaped osteons. Cement lines can be found at the interface of osteons and interstitial lamellae.

2) Circumferential lamellae - these are circular lamellae found on the external and internal surfaces of compact osseous tissue. In bone organs, the outer circumfer-

ential lamellae are found subjacent to the periosteum while inner circumferential lamellae are found adjacent to the endosteum. These lamellae are roughly perpendicular in their orientation to the lamellae associated with the underlying osteons.

CORTICAL BONE

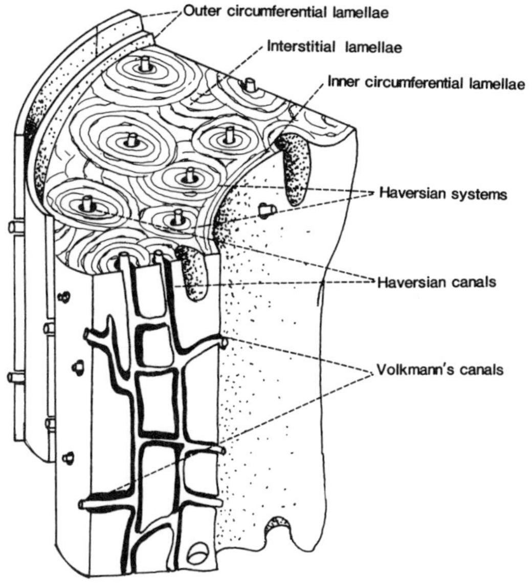

Outer circumferential lamellae
Interstitial lamellae
Inner circumferential lamellae
Haversian systems
Haversian canals
Volkmann's canals

**Fig. 2.9.** Structure of the boney cortex

Developmental History of Osseous Tissue and Bone Organs

Osseous tissue, like the other connective tissues, is derived from embryologic mesenchyme. In the embryo, some bone organs (mostly in the head region) develop by what is referred to as intramembranous ossification in which osseous tissue is formed without a preexisting surface. The initial organization of the osseous tissue is that of the woven variety with a random orientation of the collagen fibers and the absence of lamellae. Once these small islands of osseous tissue are formed, a surface is produced on which subsequent formation of additional osseous tissue can occur by apposition. It should be noted and appreciated that the term intramembranous ossification describes a transient developmental event and that the subsequent development and remodeling which occurs results in a histologic structure that is common to all bones regardless of their embryologic derivation.

In the previous form of osteogenesis, a preexisting, highly vascularized mesenchymal model or "membrane" that initially contained no surfaces was utilized for subsequent bone formation.

An alternate form in which preexisting cartilage models of bones serve a similar purpose, but in which surfaces of calcified cartilaginous tissue are available before the initiation of ossification, is referred to as endochondral (intracartilaginous) ossification. Bones that form by this mechanism are called endochondral bones and include those of the extremities, pelvis, vertebral column and base of the skull. Although the term endochondral ossification also describes a transient embryologic event, some bones formed by this mechanism retain portions of the original embryonic cartilaginous model as:

1) Articular cartilage and

2) Epiphyseal growth plates.

The function of the articular cartilage is to provide a surface of resiliency and reduced friction allowing smooth, buffered articulation with other bones at their joints. In bones with a "membrane" history, cartilage tissue within an articular surface, if present, forms after the initiation of ossification and is referred to as secondary cartilage. The epiphyseal growth plates of endochrondral bones persist during the growth period of bone organs where they serve as cartilaginous models providing a calcified cartilaginous surface necessary for bone growth. Secondary cartilage formed in membranes bones (i.e. mandible) may provide an articular surface and also act as a growth area.

## Growth of Bone Organs

Growth of bone organs occurs only by appositional growth and is effected by the initial formation of osseous tissue with a woven organization along preexisting surfaces which is later converted into a lamellar or trabecular configuration by subsequent remodeling.

Since growth of bones is totally appositional, it is obvious that the growth and maintenance of bone organs requires the presence of a surface onto which osseous tissue can be apposed. Functionally critical surfaces (envelopes) include:

1) Periosteal - subjacent to the periosteum.

2) Haversian or osteonal - lining haversian canals.

3) Cortical endosteal - adjacent to compact osseous tissue within the medullary cavity.

4) Trabecular endosteal - adjacent to trabeculae within the medullary cavity.

Increase in diameter of bone is largely dependent on the addition of osseous tissue at the periosteal surfaces. The other surfaces are important in bone modeling to meet the changing demands and stresses that a bone organ encounters during its vital period.

Increase in length is depends on endochondral growth which occurs at the epiphyseal-metaphyseal complex of long bones. It is dependent upon the presence and proper function of the epiphyseal growth plate. Its specific functions include:

1) Bone elongation and

2) Provision of a scaffolding for the appositional growth of trabeculae within the metaphysis.

The five morphologic zones of the epiphyseal plate indicative of longitudinal bone growth are:

1) Zone of resting cartilage, few small, flattened chondrocytes.

2) Zone of proliferation, division of chondrocytes resulting in interstitial growth (of the plate cartilage) in the longitudinal axis.

3) Zone of maturation, continued growth and chondrocyte maturation.

4) Zone of hypertrophy, chondrocytes are hypertrophic and regressive changes begin.

5) Zone of provisional calcification, the matrix calcifies and the chondrocytes die. The calcified cartilage provides a scaffold (surface) for the organization of trabecular osseous tissue.

The remainder of the epiphyseal-metaphyseal complex consists of the primary spongiosa (basal bony trabeculae) which is highly vascularized. The fate of the bony trabeculae of the primary spongiosa may include:

1) Replacement - the woven osseous tissue is replaced by lamellar osseous tissue.

2) Removal - shaping of the marrow cavity, or

3) Conversion - compaction resulting in generation of primary haversian systems which become part of the cortex.

## Reticular Connective Tissue

Reticular connective tissue is a highly specialized connective tissue but the same basic elements found in all other types are present in it as well, namely, cells, fibers and ground substance. Unlike cartilaginous tissue, where the ground substance is the specialized component, or osseous tissue, in which the fibers are structurally and functionally paramount, in reticular connective tissue, the cells are the predominant component. The fibers and ground substance make only minimally structural contributions.

The fundamental cell type of reticular connective tissue is the reticulum cell, which probably represents a modified fibroblast. There is evidence that the reticulum cell also possesses phagocytic properties especially for antigens and may be functionally important in certain immune-related phenomena (antigen trapping, concentration and presentation to other cells of the immune system). The reticulum cell forms a three-dimensional cellular network and produces thin collagen fibers (reticular fibers) composed of Type III collagen which in turn reinforces the structure of the cellular reticulum. The role of reticular connective tissue is largely to provide a structural framework (fibrocellular reticulum) and microenvironment conducive to formation of all types of blood cells whose precursors (CFUs or colony-forming units) inhabit it. The CFU represents an undifferentiated and pluripotent stem cell capable of differentiating in the direction of either the myeloid or lymphoid cell lines (unitarian or monophyletic theory). The location of reticular connective tissue is in areas where blood cells are normally being formed, such as the bone marrow, spleen and lymph nodes, etc. Some of these sites are the predominate location for the production of specific cell types. Thus, there are two broad categories of reticular connective tissue. They are classified by the morphologic appearance of the developmental stages of blood cells that they contain and by the mature cell types or cellular products that are produced there. It should be noted that the basic structure of the reticular connective tissue is constant but the cell types that develop within its interstices vary.

1) Myeloid tissue - this descriptive term defines the type of reticular connective tissue which contains the developmental stages of erythrocytes, granular leukocytes, monocytes and platelets. Normally, in adults, its presence is restricted to the bone marrow. NOTE: All blood cells have a history related at some point to the bone marrow. For example, the stem cells for both T and B lymphocytes originate there.

2) Lymphoid tissue - this term describes notable collections of lymphocytes and usually refers to diffuse or nodular aggregates of lymphocytes in areolar connective tissue. It may at times be used to designate the lymphocyte-packed reticular connective tissue of the lymphoid organs. The lymphoid organs will be discussed in more detail in a subsequent section on the immune system.

## Myeloid Tissue

The terms myeloid tissue and red bone marrow are often used interchangeably. It represents a form of reticular connective tissue in which the developmental stages and precirculatory forms of erythrocytes, granular leukocytes, monocytes and platelets may be found. Lymphocytes may be present as well but normally in small numbers and not usually in aggregates. The reticular fibers can not be visualized unless special techniques (silver staining) are utilized. The ground substance is so minute in quantity that it is difficult to demonstrate. The chief characteristic of myeloid tissue is the associated presence of hematopoietic elements.

## Hematopoiesis

It is convenient to study the developmental stages of bone marrow derived blood cells and their circulating mature forms in conjunction with a discussion of reticular connective tissue. Since the differentiation of the cell lines and developmental stages of blood cells is largely based on discrete morphologic properties which include minor tinctorial differences, it is appropriate to consult sources in which color plates can be found in conjunction with study of hematopoiesis. It is appropriate here to review the nomenclature of the various developmental forms in each of the cell lines. For each, the CFU is the starting point. All the developmental forms may be found in bone marrow but those that may normally circulate in the peripheral blood are marked with an asterisk (*). The successive forms are listed in increasing order of maturity and are separated from each other by a \\.

1) <u>Erythrocytic series</u> - CFU \\ proerythroblast \\ basophilic erythroblast \\ polychromatophilic erythroblast \\ orthochromatophilic erythroblast \\ reticulocyte* \\ erythrocyte*. NOTE: the reticulocyte can only be demonstrated in peripheral blood with special staining techniques and is normally present in small numbers. Increased numbers can signify a disease state. Orthochromatophilic erythroblasts are also known as normoblasts.

2) <u>Granulocytic series</u> - CFU \\ myeloblast \\ promyelocyte \\ myelocyte \\ metamyelocyte \\ polymorphonuclear leukocyte* NOTE: From the myelocyte stage on, specific cytoplasmic granules are present that allow subclassification into basophilic, eosinophilic or neutrophilic types. An intermediate stage between the metamyelocyte stage and PMN stage of neutrophils known as the band or stab occurs and a small number of these can be observed normally in the peripheral blood. An increase in their number is considered pathological.

3) <u>Megakaryocytic series</u> - CFU \\ megakaryoblast \\ metamegakaryocyte \\ megakaryocyte \\ platelets* NOTE: platelets are also known as thrombocytes and are anuclear cytoplasmic derivatives of the megakaryocyte.

4) <u>Monocytic series</u> - CFU \\ promonocyte \\ monocyte* NOTE: monocytes that leave the blood to reside in the connective tissues or organs (i.e. lung alveoli) are termed macrophages (histiocytes).

## <u>Formed Elements of the Blood</u>

The peripheral blood contains certain formed elements, most of which originate within the reticular connective tissue of the bone marrow. Following their formation, they are released as mature circulating cells or cellular-derived elements. These include erythrocytes, platelets, granulocytes (neutrophils, eosinophils and basophils) and agranulocytes (monocytes and lymphocytes). Although some of the circulating lymphocytes have an immediate bone-marrow origin, most of them are recirculating between lymphoid organs (spleen and lymph nodes) and the connective tissue compartment. Platelets and erythrocytes are not bonafide cells because they are anuclear but both have a cellular origin in the bone marrow.

1) Erythrocytes - these appear as anucleate, biconcave disks measuring approximately 7.5 microns in diameter. Intracytoplasmic organelles are largely lacking. Instead the cytoplasmic content consists almost entirely of molecules of hemoglobin which imparts a reddish coloration. Although erythrocytes are incapable of protein synthesis, slightly immature forms (reticulocytes) contain some residual RNA demonstrable by supravital staining. Their average lifespan in the peripheral blood is approximately 120 days.

2) Platelets - these are the smallest formed elements of the blood (2-4 microns in length) appearing as flattened, convex disks. By light microscopy, two regions are apparent, the granulomere and the hyalomere. As its name implies the granulomere is a central zone containing granules which can be seen in traditionally stained blood smears. Three types of granules are present which can be differentiated in electron micrographs: dense granules, alpha granules and lysosomes. Dense granules contain serotonin, ADP, ATP and calcium while the content of alpha granules includes various platelet-derived clotting factors. The outer zone or hyalomere is homogeneous, pale-staining and contains cytoskeletal elements.

3) Neutrophils - also known as polymorphonuclear leukocytes because the nucleus is normally multilobed. The nuclei of most circulating neutrophils contain 3 to 5 lobes connected by thin condensed chromatin strands. A few nonsegmented "band" forms may also be observed which indicates a less mature state. As maturation of the cell occurs, its nucleus becomes progressively more lobulated. In the female, additional condensed chromatin may be seen in the form of a "drumstick" extending from one of the lobes. It represents the inactivated X chromosome and is the homologue of the Barr body present in other cells. The specific granules of neutrophils stain light pink in standard blood preparations. Primary (azurophilic) granules, fewer but larger in size, are present as well. The latter are largely lysosomal in nature. Neutrophils are intensely phagocytic toward particulate material especially bacteria. Like other granulocytes they have a relatively brief life span of about 3 to 7 days.

4) Eosinophils - these are bilobed cells containing large, red-staining cytoplasmic granules. Eosinophils contain antihistaminic substances which play a role in the control of immune-related and allergic responses and a major basic protein important in killing of certain extracellular parasites.

5) Basophils - represent the smallest number of circulating blood cells. The nucleus, if observable, is nonsegmented or bilobed. Its presence is often obscured by many large, dark-staining specific granules. The granules contain heparin as well as other substances.

6) Monocytes - these contain a kidney-shaped nucleus which contains a delicate network of extended chromatin. The cytoplasm is extensive and may contain a few azurophilic granules (primary lysosomes). In the blood, monocytes are functionally immature but once they establish residence in connective tissue or organs they become actively phagocytic. Their life span may be up to several months.

7) Lymphocytes - the nucleus of these cells is usually round and quite densely stained. The cytoplasm stains basophilic and varies in amount from a scant rim around the nucleus to an amount approaching that of monocytes. The life span is highly variable but some lymphocytes may exist for several years. Morphologically, a distinction can not be made between T and B lymphocytes in standard stained preparations.

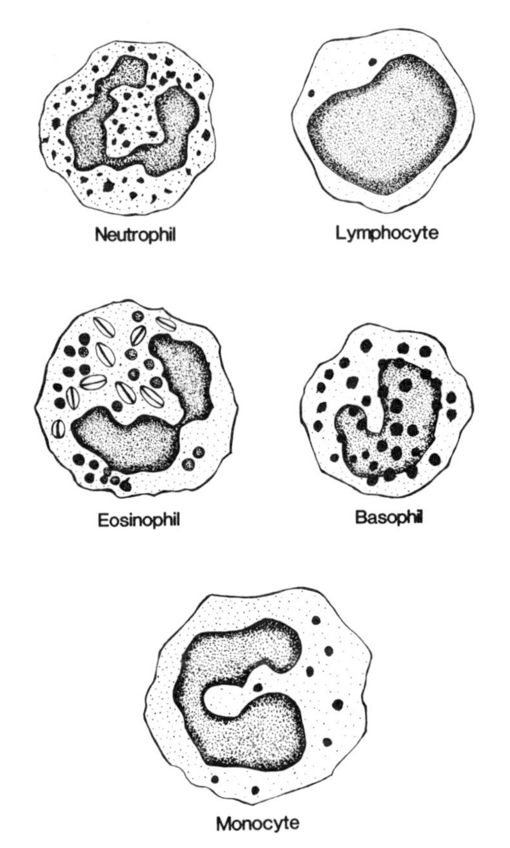


**Fig. 2.10.** Formed elements of the peripheral blood

## MUSCULAR TISSUE

Functionally there are two categories of muscle tissue, voluntary and involuntary, dependent upon whether they are controlled by the central nervous system or autonomic nervous system, respectively. Morphologically, three types of muscular tissue are recognized: smooth, cardiac and skeletal. The first two are involuntary while the latter is usually but not invariably voluntary. In common, they synthesize and maintain an intracellular component of filamentous proteins whose interactions result in cells or fibers that possess a high degree of contractile specialization. Although many other cell types are capable of producing contractile events (cell motility, alteration of cell shape), those comprising muscle tissue are structurally differentiated to emphasize the property of contractility to the point that it is their primary functional role.

Skeletal muscle fibers and cardiac muscle cells have a distinctive banded appearance when observed in a longitudinal orientation under the light microscope. This visual property is due to a highly-ordered arrangement of intrasarcoplasmic contractile protein filaments. As a result, skeletal and cardiac muscle are sometimes collectively referred to as striated muscle. The cells of smooth muscle, as the name implies, do not show the characteristic transverse bands (cross-striations) because the filamentous contractile proteins which they contain lack the regular geometric configuration present in the striated variety.

Although actin (a thin filament) and myosin (a thick filament) are found in many other cell types, they are the major intracellular proteins of muscle cells. Actin is a 42,000 Dalton protein present in a globular form, G-actin, which is capable of polymerizing into a filamentous form, F-actin. In striated muscle cells or fibers, F-actin is the major form present. Associated with the actin filaments are a variety of regulatory proteins including troponin and tropomyosin. Myosin molecules have a molecular weight of 470,000 Daltons and are composed of heavy meromyosin and light meromyosin. Heavy meromyosin possesses a globular head and ATPase activity.

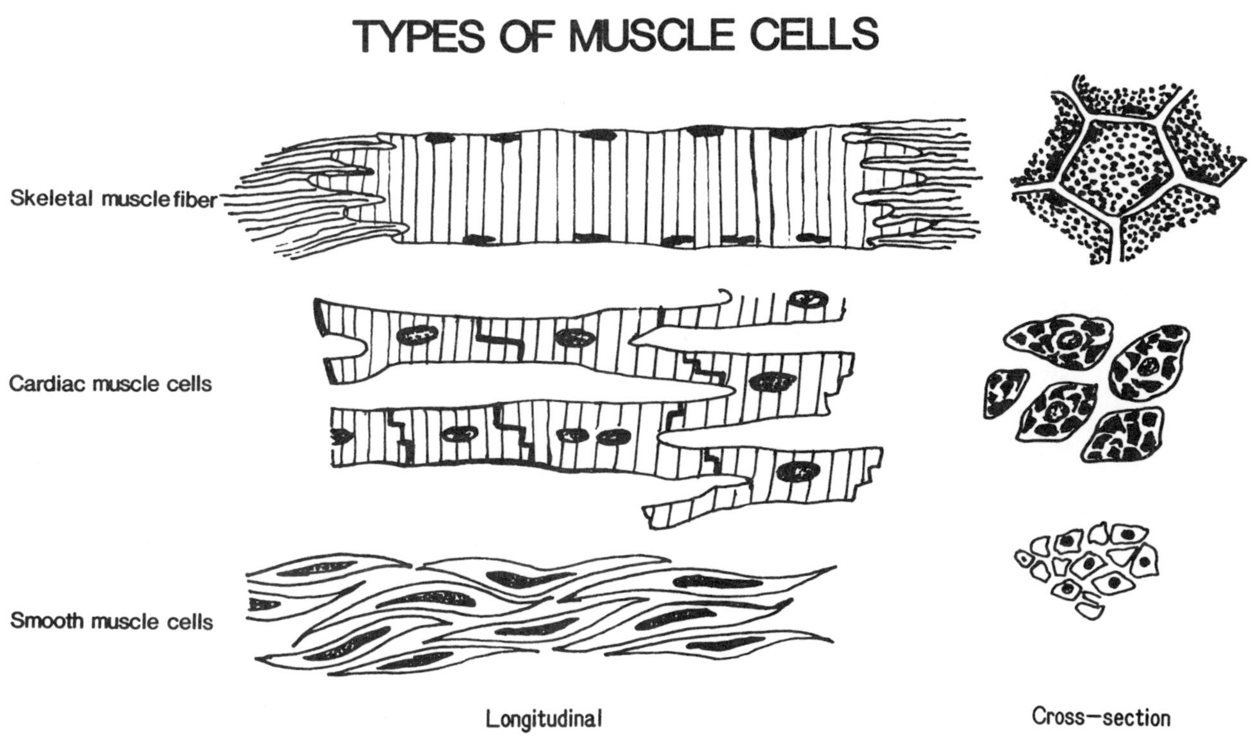


**Fig. 2.11.** Cells and fibers of the three types of muscle tissue

## Smooth Muscle

Smooth muscle cells, for the most part, have a mesodermal origin from embryonic mesenchyme. Notable exceptions are the ectodermally-derived smooth muscle of the nipple, scrotum and iridic muscle of the eye. The contractile myoepithelial cells of various glands are also of ectodermal origin and are contained within the basal lamina of the gland epithelia.

The major contractile filaments, myosin and actin are present but are not organized into bundles (myofibrils) so that the sarcoplasm has a homogeneous appearance at the light microscopic level. The cells, are small and fusiform (spindle-shaped) and contain a single elongate, centrally placed nucleus in which one or more nucleoli can usually be observed. In longitudinal view, the nucleus may appear straight, folded, pleated or spiral depending on the contractile state of the cell at the time of tissue fixation.

The following key points are worth considering:

1) Smooth muscles cells may be found occasionally as isolated single cells but are more frequently arranged in sheets or layers around tubular structures such as the gut or blood vessels.

2) Other locations include the myometrium of the uterus, muscular wall of the urinary bladder and ureters, arrector pili muscle of certain hairs and walls of respiratory passages.

3) When present in bundles, they are arranged in a staggered orientation so that cross-sections through a bundle in a single plane produces numerous round profiles of varying size. Depending on whether the cut passes near the longitudinal center of the cell determines if the individual cross-sectional profile will contain a central nucleus or not.

4) Ultrastructurally, the cells are contained within external basal laminae, the sarcoplasmic reticulum is composed of long tubular elements and T (transverse) tubules are lacking.

5) Innervation is by nonmyelinated postganglionic fibers of both limbs of the autonomic nervous system but a one to one relationship of nerve ending to muscle is not present. Smooth muscle cells can be hormonally evoked to contract or in some cases contraction can be elicited by physical stretch.

6) Gap junctions may be present between adjacent cells.

## Cardiac Muscle

Cardiac muscle cells contain a single (rarely two) centrally placed nucleus and are structurally characterized by their frequent branching. The cells are connected end to end at special sites referred to as intercalated disks. Cardiac muscle cells are striated as are skeletal muscle fibers but the above characteristics differentiate the two at the light microscopic level. Cardiac muscle is restricted in location to the myocardium of the heart and proximal portions of the aorta, venae cavae and pulmonary vessels. Other important features of cardiac muscle tissue include:

1) Myosin and actin filaments are arranged parallel to each other in bundles known as myofibrils.

2) The regular arrangement of actin and myosin filaments is responsible for the cross-banded appearance.

3) Myofibrils are composed of numerous subunits known as sarcomeres, the functional units of striated muscle.

4) The length of the sarcomere depends upon it state of contraction.

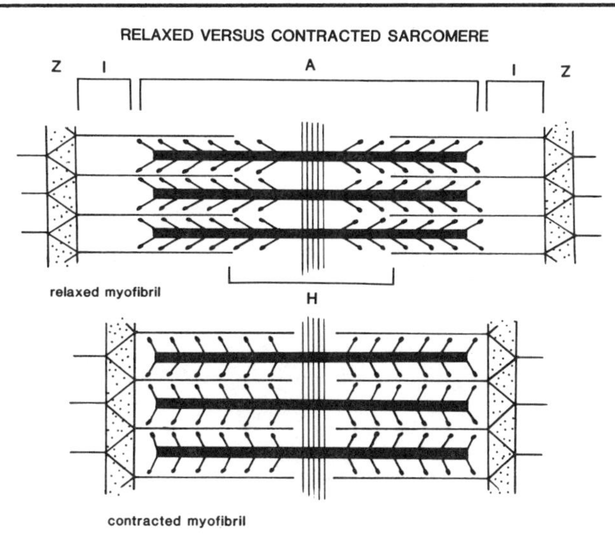


**Fig. 2.12.** Change in sarcomeric length with contraction

5) Ultrastructurally, individual sarcomeres exhibit a number of bands and lines. They are delimited at both ends by the Z line or disk. The central, darkest

region includes the length of myosin filaments and is known as the A band. Actin filaments are also present within the A band except in a lighter central region, the H band. In the middle of the H band the myosin molecules are thickest at the M line. The ends of the sarcomere containing only actin filaments constitutes part of another light band, the I band. A complete I band consists of the ends of two contiguous sarcomeres and the centrally placed Z line. During contraction, the sarcomeres (but not the individual filaments) decrease in length. This is due to an increase in the region of overlap of the actin and myosin filaments. Correspondingly, there is a decrease in the length of the H and I bands but the A band remains unchanged.

6) The intercalated disks of light microscopy are located at the Z disks and in electron micrographs are seen to consist of three structurally distinct regions: the macula adherens (desmosome), the fascia adherens and the gap junction. Tubules (T tubules) are present at the Z lines.

7) Regions in which a terminal cistern of the sarcoplasmic reticulum (SR) is associated with the T tubule are known as diads. Although the membranes of the T tubule and SR are only closely apposed, peculiar structures known as junctional feet span the space between the two. This area of structural specialization is thought to play a role in triggering release of stored calcium ions in the SR brought about by the depolarization of the T tubule. Functionally similar "diad-like" structures occur between the terminal cisterns of the SR and sarcolemma.

8) Specialized cardiac muscle cells known as Purkinje fibers are found as components of the conduction system of the heart. They are structurally and functionally modified not for contraction but for distribution of the impulse for contraction throughout the heart. In sections viewed by light microscopy, the Purkinje fibers stain lighter than do regular cardiac muscle cells and are thicker in diameter. They contain only a few myofibrils, lack T tubules and are not connected with each other at typical intercalated disks but gap junctions and desmosomes are present between the cells.

9) Cardiac muscle is innervated by both limbs of the autonomic nervous system. Unmyelinated fibers containing synaptic vesicles appose the sarcolemma but are not associated with a postsynaptic motor end plate as found in skeletal muscle fibers.

## Skeletal Muscle

Skeletal muscle fibers are a syncytium formed by the fusion of numerous myoblasts and as a result are multinucleated. The nuclei are located in a peripheral position just below the sarcolemma. Actin and myosin filaments are aligned as they are in cardiac muscle so that cross-striations are present. Myofilaments are oriented into parallel bundles known as myofibrils which are composed of sarcomeres arranged end to end along the horizontal axis of the myofiber. Numerous myofibrils comprise an individual myofiber. Each myofiber is covered externally by its sarcolemma, a basal lamina and a delicate layer of connective tissue, the endomysium, which binds it to neighboring myofibers.

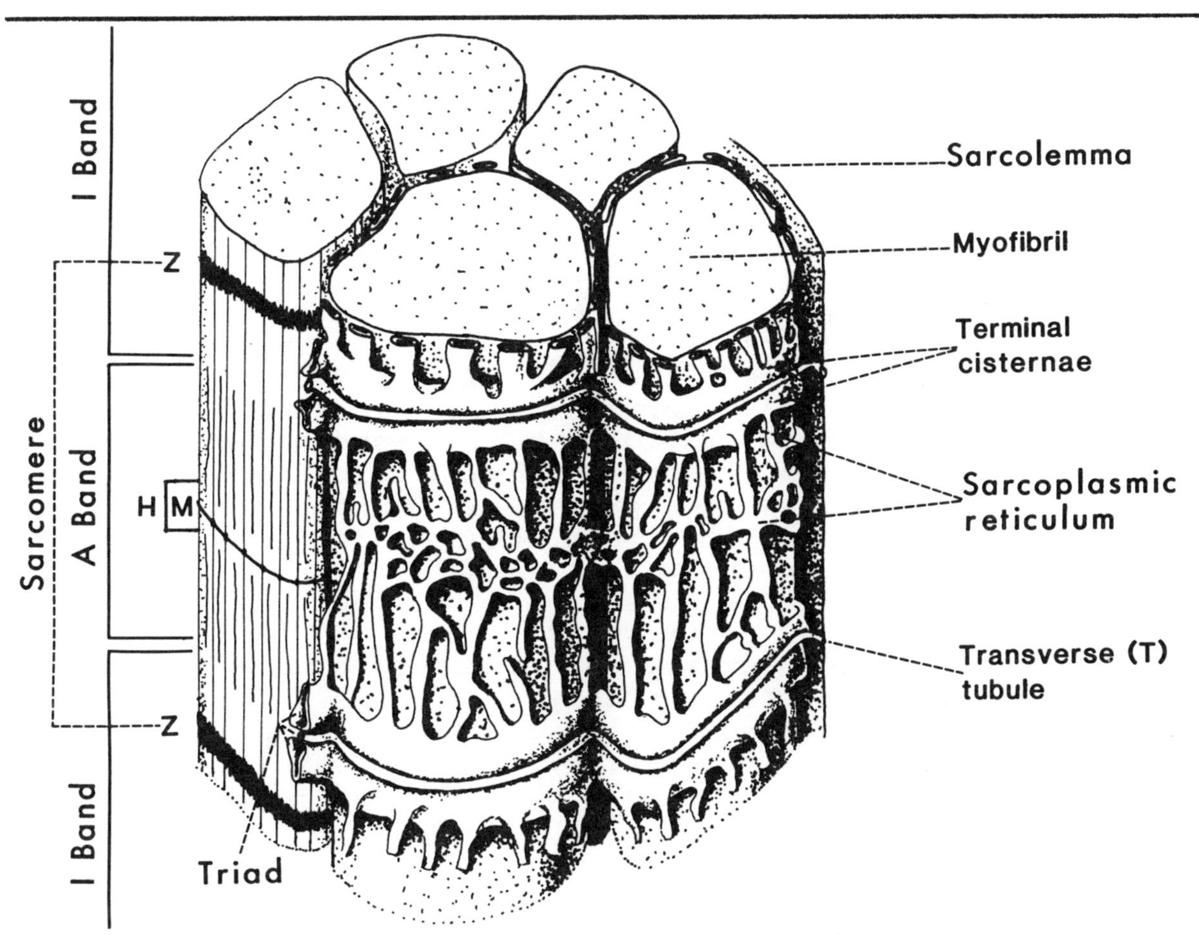


**Fig. 2.13.** Ultrastructural features of skeletal myofibers

Adjacent groups of myofibers are gathered into bundles or fascicles by a connective tissue investment, the perimysium. Finally, the gross muscle consists of several to many fascicles bound together by a dense fibrous sheath, the epimysium or deep fascia. Other key points include:

1) Each myofibril is irregularly circumscribed by the sarcoplasmic reticulum.

2) Transversely oriented invaginations of the sarcolemma, T tubules, are smaller but more frequent in skeletal than in cardiac muscle. In skeletal muscle, the T tubules are located at the junctions of the A and I bands and are apposed on each side by terminal cisterns of the sarcoplasmic reticulum. This morphologic arrangement may be observed in electron micrographs as structures known as triads.

3) The structural integrity and function of skeletal muscle is dependent on innervation by lower motor neurons. Loss of innervation results in degradation of contractile proteins, atrophy and eventual loss of the denervated myofiber. Neural influence on skeletal myofibers by lower motor neurons induces structural, metabolic and functional modifications so that a variety of different fiber types exist in mature muscle. Two major populations of myofibers occur in the human referred to as Type I and Type II. They are differentiated physiologically by their speed and duration of contraction. Type I myofibers contract slowly but are capable of sustained contraction (slow-twitch fibers) whereas those classified as Type II contract more rapidly but for shorter periods (fast-twitch fibers). These physiologic features correlate roughly with the predominate metabolic pathways for energy production and thus with the biochemical components found within each type. As a result, the different fiber types can be identified with certain histochemical techniques. Although a great number of these procedures may be utilized to distinguish fiber types, the most commonly used ones demonstrate either myosin ATPase, oxidative or glycolytic enzymes. Type I fibers possess relatively less myosin ATPase activity (demonstrated at alkaline pH) but greater activity of oxidative enzymes. Correspondingly, there are greater numbers of mitochondria and more myoglobin present in these fibers. Type II fibers exhibit greater activity of glycolytic enzymes, less mitochondria, less myoglobin but more glycogen stores.

It should be emphasized that human muscles consist of a random mixture of the two main types of myofibers. This is unlike some lower animals in which whole muscles or large parts of a muscle may be composed of myofibers of the same type. It should also be noted that all myofibers within the same motor unit (innervated by the same lower motor neuron) are of identical type but are haphazardly dispersed throughout the fascicle.

4) The site of neuromuscular transmission in skeletal muscle is known as the motor end plate. This is a structurally specialized region which includes contributions by the axon terminal of the lower motor neuron, a nonmyelinating Schwann cell and the sarcolemma of the myofiber. The sarcolemma of the myofiber in the region of the motor end plate is depressed below the surface of the surrounding plasmalemma. This depression or trough is occupied by the axon terminal and is called the primary synaptic cleft (PSC). Within the base of the primary cleft, numerous complex invaginations of the plasmalemma (junctional folds) are present constituting the secondary synaptic clefts (SSC). The primary and secondary synaptic clefts comprise the sole plate of the sarcolemma. Acetylcholine receptors are located along the outer aspects of the SSC whereas acetylcholinesterase is located in the depths of the SSC. The external basal lamina of the myofibers intervenes between the axon terminal of the innervating neuron and the sole plate. The neuromuscular junction is covered externally by a nonmyelinating Schwann cell. Acetylcholine-containing synaptic vesicles are present within the axoplasm of the axon terminal.

## NERVOUS TISSUE

Nervous tissue has an ectodermal origin and therefore displays many features of epithelia. The cells are closely arranged, little extracellular space is present and specialized junctions occur between many of the cells. The cells of the nervous tissues fall into two categories. The functional nerve cells or neurons are highly specialized for the property of excitability. They are capable of receiving and transmitting information in the form of neural impulses. The other cells of nervous tissue are supportive in their function and are necessary to establish an environment in which the neurons can achieve their function in an efficient manner. These cells are collectively referred to as glia and with one exception are also ectodermal in origin. The main mass of neural tissue is located in the organs of the central nervous system (CNS) where it comprises the vast majority of the tissue of the cerebrum, cerebellum and spinal cord. Since virtually all structures of the body are innervated, processes of nerve cells and their supporting elements are observed outside the CNS as well. In aggregate, these components comprise what is known as the peripheral nervous system (PNS). The present discussion will concentrate on the elements and functional features of nervous tissue rather than on the interaction with other tissues and their composite organization into nervous organs.

## Cells of Nervous Tissue

The nerve cells or neurons are diverse in structure but have in common the property of excitability. They are capable of propagating and conducting a nervous impulse and of communicating with other neurons or with effector cells by means of a specialized cellular junction termed a synapse.

The supporting cells or glia display intimate structural contact with neurons. Glia, like neurons, possess one or more attenuated cytoplasmic processes but, unlike them, are not specialized for excitability.

### Neurons

The neuron consists of a cell body called the soma or perikaryon and few to many attenuated cytoplasmic processes which radiate out from the cell body. Depending upon their functional role these processes are termed axons or dendrites. Because of these peripheral processes, neuronal structure is highly diversified and some neurons may be more than a meter in length.

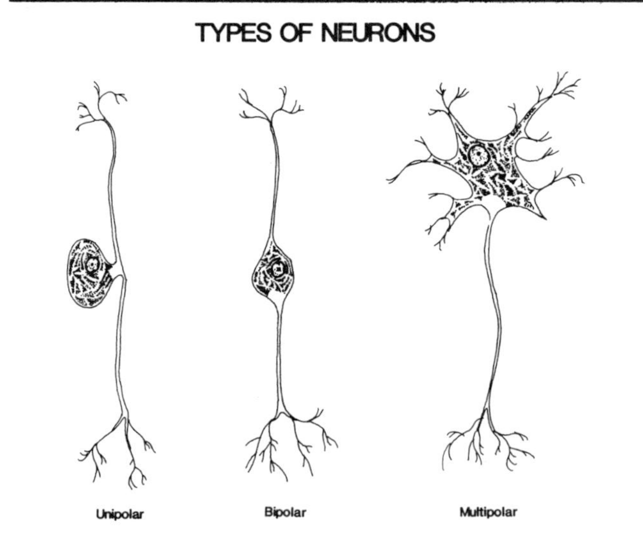


**Fig. 2.14.** Basic types of neurons (Courtesy Dr. R. Snell)

Neurons may be classified by their shape which is due largely to the appearance and location of their axons and dendrites. Four basic forms of neurons are recognized:

1) Multipolar neurons - these possess many processes including an axon and many dendrites. Most motor

neurons are multipolar but not all multipolar neurons are motor.

2) Bipolar neurons - as their name implies these neurons possess two processes arising at opposite poles of the cell. One functions as an axon, the other as a dendrite. Typically they are associated with special sense reception such as olfaction, hearing and balance.

3) Unipolar neurons - these cells are round to oval and possess a single process which divides a short distance from the cell body into a functional dendrite and axon. Unipolar neurons are sensory or afferent in function and are found in the sensory ganglia of spinal and some cranial nerves.

4) Anaxonic neurons - as implied by the name, these lack an axon so that both receptor and effector function is carried out by dendrites. An example of these are the amacrine cells of the inner cell layer of the retina.

The soma or cell body contains the cytoplasm (perikaryon) and the nucleus. The perikaryon varies in shape depending on the type of neuron (multipolar, bipolar, unipolar). The size is considerably variable ranging from the very small granule cells of the cerebellum (4 microns) to the large multipolar lower motor neurons in the anterior gray columns of the spinal cord (140 microns). The perikaryon of the neuron contains most of the organelles found in other cells and in certain regions of the CNS a pigment termed neuromelanin may be present. Neuromelanin may be found within certain neurons of the olfactory bulb, locus ceruleus in the floor of the fourth ventricle, substantia nigra of the midbrain and the reticular formation. Because neurons are part of the permanent cell population, they may also store lipofuscin in increasing amounts with advancing age.

The perikaryon of many, but not all, neurons contains so-called Nissl substance. This intracytoplasmic material is best demonstrated with basic aniline dyes where it appears as variously shaped clumps of small granules. It may be observed in the perikaryon and proximal portions of dendrites but, for the most part, is absent from the axon including its most proximal portion, the axon hillock. By electron microscopy, Nissl substance corresponds to clusters of RER and free ribosomes, the latter of which are oriented into linear arrays.

Other features of the perikaryon include the presence of subsurface cisternae, microtubules and microfilaments. In neurons and certain glia, microfilaments are called neurofilaments. They are morphologically similar to intermediate filaments but are chemically distinct. With metal impregnation techniques bundles of neurofilaments (neurofibrils) may be demonstrated. Mitochondria are usually quite numerous and a prominent Golgi apparatus may be observed.

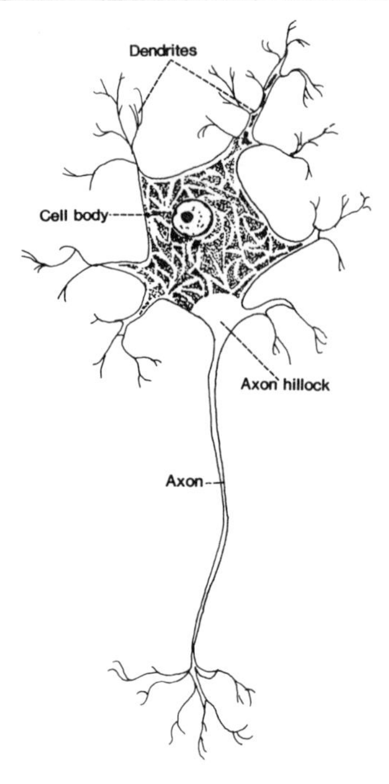


**Fig. 2.15.** The neuron (Courtesy Dr. R. Snell)

The nucleus of most neurons is spherical in shape and thus appears round in tissue sections. It often has a striking appearance with an open chromatin pattern and a prominent and relatively large nucleolus. In most neurons, it is centrally located. Exceptions to this are the eccentrically placed nuclei of the motor neurons in the autonomic ganglia of the PNS.

Radiating out from the perikaryon are various types and numbers of cell processes. Usually present is a single axon and one or more dendrites. Dendrites are the receptor portion of the neuron and convey information toward the cell body. They are usually but not always shorter than the axon. Dendrites often branch repeatedly and present a surface studded with small spines or knobs (dendritic spines or gemmules). The proximal dendrite may contain Nissl substance and therefore is a site of protein synthesis. Other contents of the dendrite are microtubules, neurofilaments and mitochondria.

The axon or axis cylinder may arise from the perikaryon or proximal portion of a dendrite. It acts as the effector portion of the neuron and conveys neural impulses away from the cell body. The point of emergence of the axon is represented by a conical area known as the axon hillock. Axons may give off collaterals and in their terminal portions may be quite branched. The plasmalemma covering the axis cylinder is often referred to as the axolemma and its cytoplasmic contents as the axoplasm.

Usually devoid of Nissl substance, and therefore unable to synthesize protein locally, the axoplasm contains mitochondria, neurofilaments and microtubules. The latter may play a role in the axoplasmic transport of proteins and other substances from their site of synthesis in the perikaryon to the far reaches of the axon.

## Synapses

The usual effect of a nervous impulse upon the neuron is the release of a special chemical from the axon terminal. These chemicals are generally referred to as neurotransmitter substances. The synapse is a region of specialized intercellular attachment between two neurons or between a neuron and an effector cell.

The axon at the site of a synapse is generally enlarged (bullous) and contains mitochondria, neurofibrillar material and clusters of synaptic vesicles in which the presumptive neurotransmitter substances are located. The axon terminal is called the presynaptic element, the cell that it contacts (another neuron or an effector cell), the postsynaptic element and the intervening intercellular space, the synaptic cleft. The membranes of the pre- and postsynaptic elements are usually modified in the area of the synapse and by electron microscopy may be coated with an electron dense material.

Neuron to neuron synapses are classified by the location of the synapse on the postsynaptic element. Thus synapses may be axodendritic, axosomatic or axoaxonic.

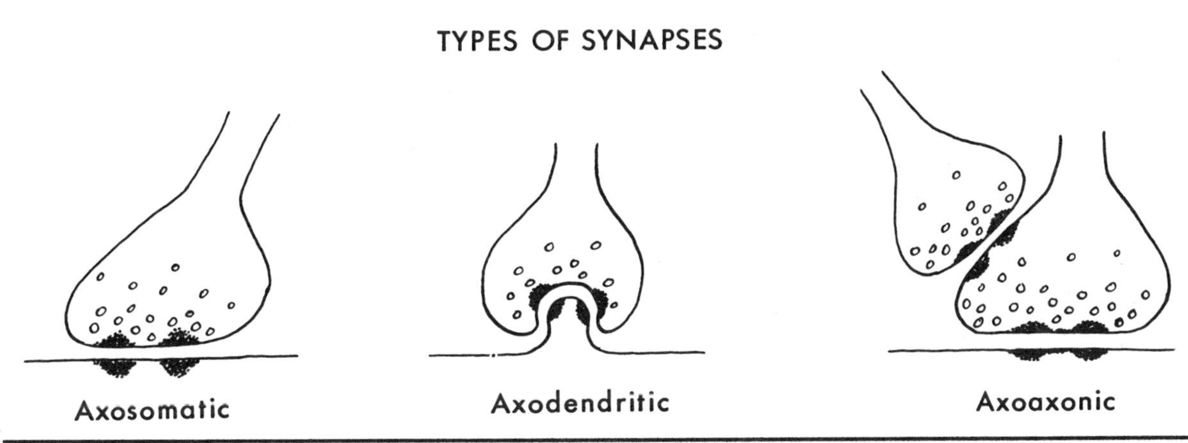


**Fig. 2.16.** Various configurations of synaptic sites

There have been a variety of biochemical substances identified that are capable of acting as neurotransmitters. Acetylcholine and norepinephrine are the ones more readily recalled but others including dopamine, serotonin, gamma-aminobutyric acid (GABA) and the more recently discovered enkephalins and endorphins are included in this category.

Membrane-bound synaptic vesicles contain or bind the neurotransmitter chemicals. The morphologic appearance of these vesicles in electron micrographs can lend a clue to the type of transmitter substance present. The vesicles of cholinergic synapses are clear while adrenergic synapses are associated with vesicles containing dense cores. It should be emphasized that not all synapses are of the chemical variety but that they predominate in the PNS and are also found within the CNS. Another type of synapse referred to as an electrical synapse occurs within the CNS. In these, a gap junction is present between the pre- and postsynaptic elements and depolarization of the postsynaptic element is mediated not by chemical substances but by ionic current.

## Neuroglia

Glia cells are found both in the CNS and PNS. In the central nervous system they consist of astrocytes, oligodendroglial cells, microglial cells and ependymal cells.

1) Astrocytes - are stellate in shape because of the presence of many cytoplasmic processes. These cells contain characteristic cytoplasmic filaments of the intermediate type and glycogen. Usually one or more peripheral processes terminate in the vicinity of blood vessels. There are two general types of astrocytes:
    a) Protoplasmic astrocytes - these are found principally in gray matter of brain and spinal cord. They may terminate on blood vessels (sucker feet) and may cover neuronal synaptic surfaces.
    b) Fibrous astrocytes - contain fewer but straighter cytoplasmic processes than the protoplasmic variety and many more bundles of neurofilaments. This type is found chiefly within the white matter and is responsible for filling in damaged areas of the neuropil through a reactive process known as gliosis.

2) Oligodendrocytes - also known as oligodendroglia. They are smaller than astrocytes and have a few small, delicate branches. Their nuclei tend to be smaller, more spherical and condensed than astrocyte nuclei. In tissue sections viewed by light microscopy they are often surrounded by a nearly unavoidable shrinkage artifact which appears as a halo around each cell. Ultrastructurally, intermediate filaments and cytoplasmic glycogen characteristic of astrocytes are absent. There are three general types of oligodendrocytes depending on their location and presumably their function:
    a) Perivascular - located around vessels.

b) Perineuronal - around neurons in gray matter.

c) Interfascicular - found within the white matter where they perform the chief function of the oligodendroglial cell population, the formation and maintenance of myelin in the CNS.

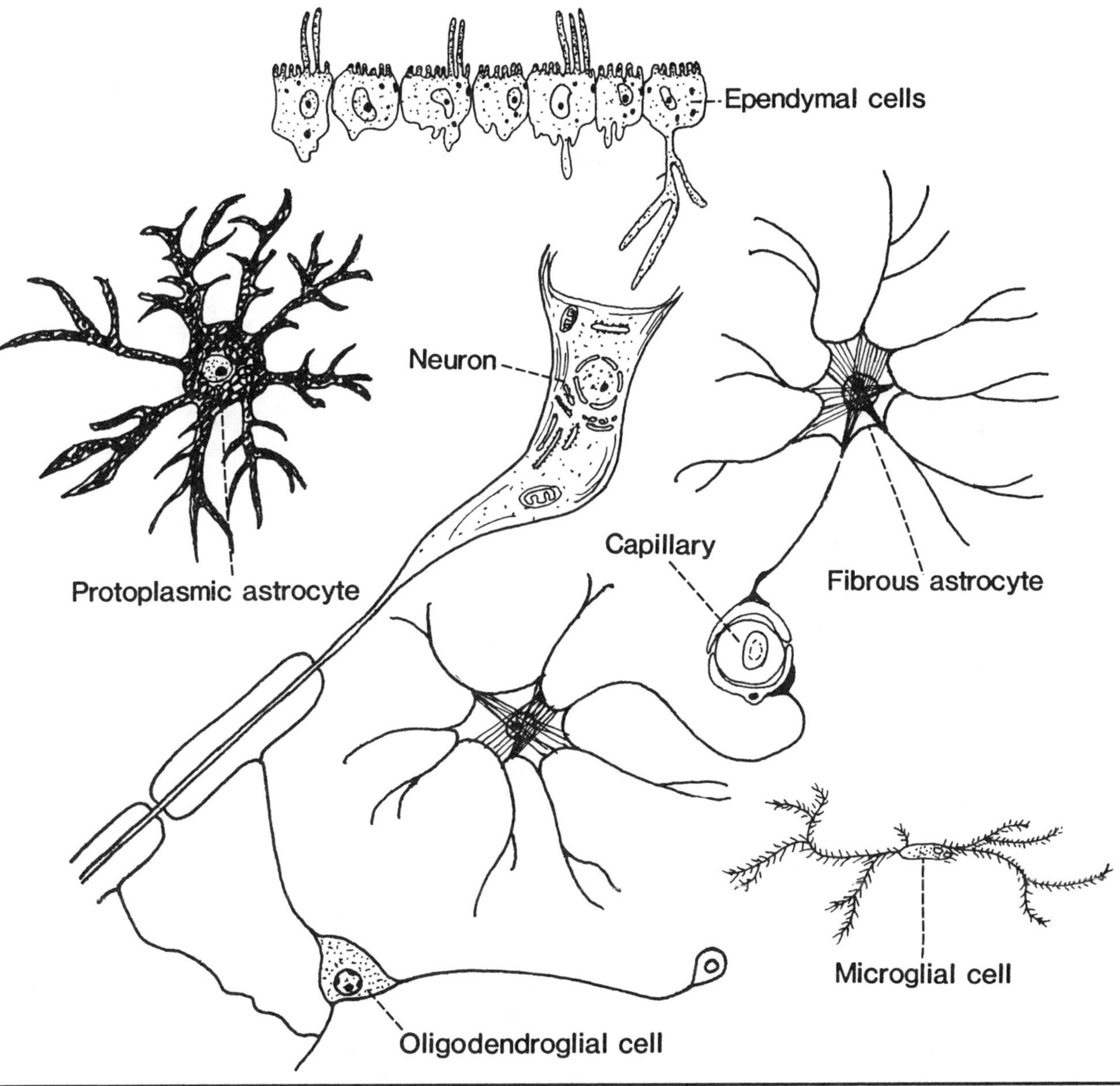


**Fig. 2.17.** Structure and relationships of CNS and PNS glia (Courtesy of Dr. R. Snell)

A key point concerning myelination of CNS axons is that one oligodendroglial cell is capable of providing the myelin sheath for a number of axons. They may also ensheathe a number of unmyelinated axons.

3) Microglia - these are said to be the only glial cell that is not of neuroectodermal origin. They are believed to be derived from blood monocytes and are thus of mesodermal origin. They comprise one component of the so-called mononuclear phagocyte system. Their function is thus one of phagocytosis and when greatly distended by ingested material they are referred to as compound granular corpuscles or more commonly as "gitter cells". When inactive they may contain a number of short processes and appear in sections viewed by routine light microscopy as small cells with ovoid, dense nuclei and are termed rod cells.

4) Ependymal cells - line the cavities of the brain and spinal cord (ventricles and central canal) and are a component of the choroid plexus. They are closely packed and appear as a simple cuboidal epithelium but are in reality the apical cells of the neural tube epithelium. They contain variable inner processes which ramify into the CNS to end on blood vessels. In certain areas during intrauterine life and for a time after birth they may display cilia on their luminal surfaces.

The glia of the peripheral nervous system include the PNS homologue of the interfascicular oligodendrocyte, the Schwann cell, and in certain PNS ganglia, the satellite cells.

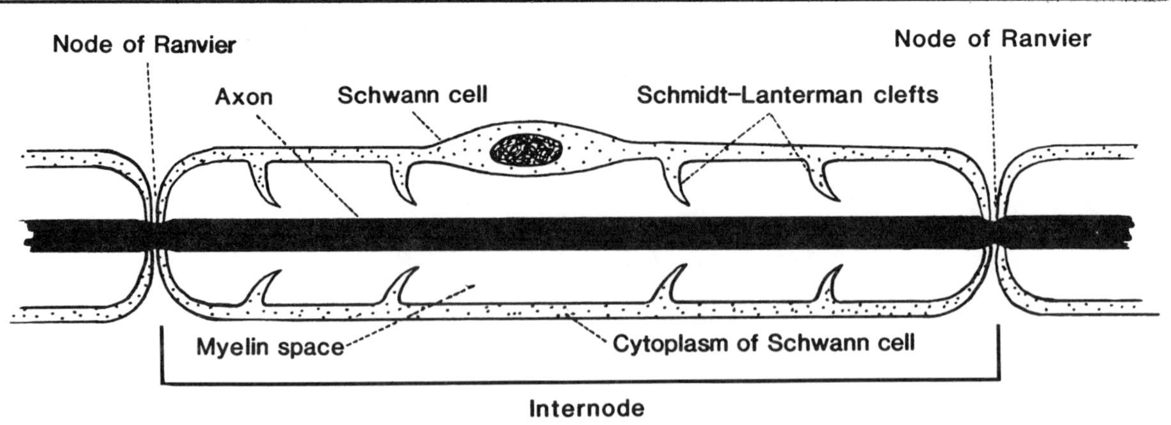


**Fig. 2.18.** Structural relationships of the Schwann cell and a myelinated axon.

1) Schwann cells - are of neural crest origin and function chiefly to provide an investment around the axons located outside the CNS.

---

SCHWANN CELL INVESTMENTS OF AXONS

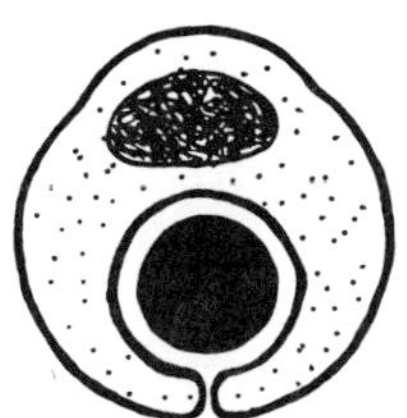

Initial stage of axonal myelination
- myelin not yet formed

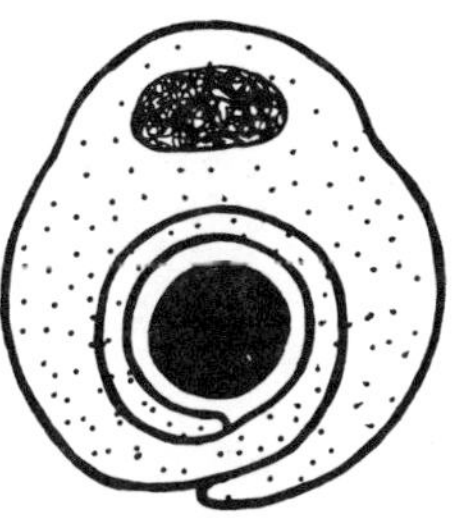

Early myelination of single axon
- few lamellae present

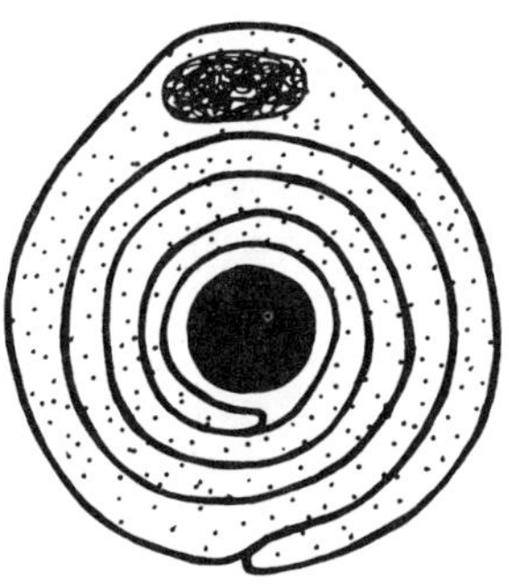

Later stage of myelination
- more lamellae added

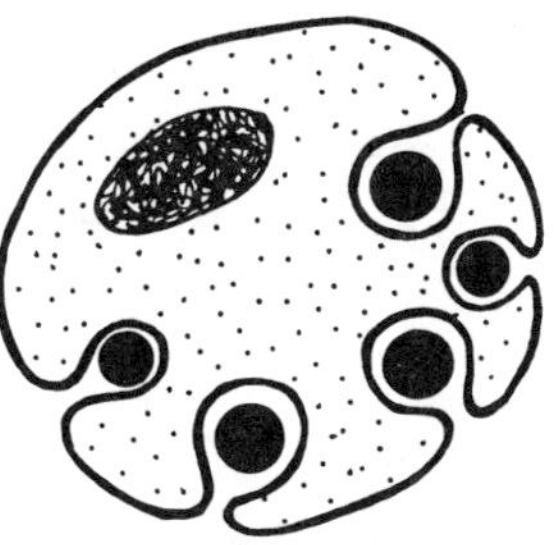

Multiple unmyelinated axons

---

**Fig. 2.19.** Relationships of Schwann cells with myelinated and unmyelinated axons

Although one Schwann cell may invest a number of unmyelinated fibers, it can contribute myelin to only one axon. Myelin consists of spirally disposed layers of Schwann cell plasma membrane that become closely apposed. It is said that myelination in the PNS occurs as a result of repeated circumnavagation of the Schwann cell about the axon so that it becomes covered by circumferetial lamellae of Schwann cell membrane. The cytoplasmic surfaces of the membrane fuse and are referred to as the major dense line when viewed at the electron microscope level. Between major dense lines

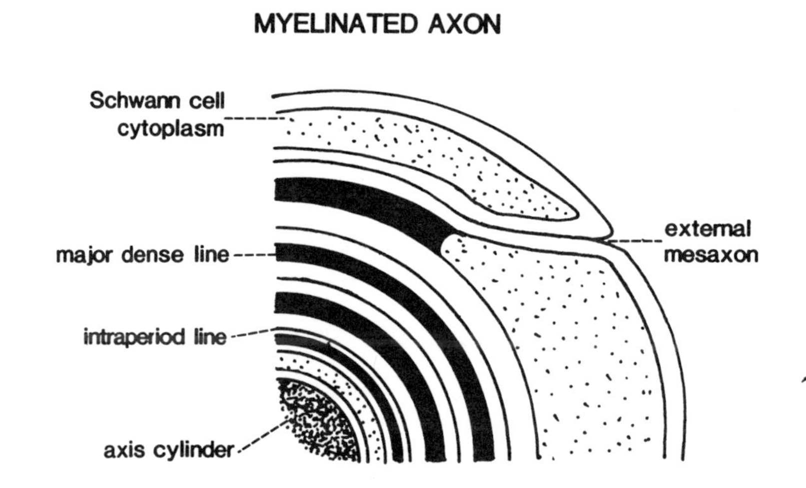


**Fig. 2.20.** Structure of myelin lamellae

are the intraperiod lines. Retention of Schwann cell cytoplasm within the myelin lamellae results in the presence of the so-called Schmidt-Lanterman clefts or incisures. The appearance of the myelin sheath differs depending on the type of fixation employed. In osmium-fixed sections oriented longitudinally, the myelin contributed by successive Schwann cells appears as sausage-shaped structures termed internodes. The breaks between internodes are called the nodes of Ranvier at which a short segment of naked axon is present. Because the osmium fixation stains the lipid of the myelin sheath black, the axon covered by it is not apparent. In routinely fixed tissue, most of the lipid of the membranes is dissolved out so that the major component of the myelin sheath is removed. Left behind is a proteinaceous residue known as neurokeratin. Careful examination of longitudinal sections of peripheral nerve will reveal the internodal outlines, the presence of neurokeratin, the location of the nodes of Ranvier and depending on the plane of section, segments of the axis cylinder.

2) Satellite cells - satellite cells are intimately associated with the neurons of peripheral ganglia. Each ganglion cell (neuron) is covered externally by a single layer of ovoid satellite cells which serve to isolate the cell body from the capillary network within the ganglion. The satellite cells are in turn covered by a basal lamina and a layer of collagen fibers and fibroblasts referred to as capsule cells. The layer of satellite cells is continuous at the axon with the Schwann cell layer. Satellite cells, like Schwann cells, are of neural crest origin.

## UNIT II: PROFICIENCY EXAM

**DIRECTIONS:** For the following questions select the one best answer which completes the statement or answers the question.

1) The epithelial surface modifications which appear to be associated with absorptive processes are:
   A. Brush or striated borders.
   B. Stereocilia.
   C. Desmosomes (macula adherens).
   D. Gap junctions.
   E. None of the above.

2) Characteristics of epithelia include:
   A. Absence of blood and lymphatic vessels.
   B. A free or unattached surface.
   C. Attachment to underlying connective tissue.
   D. Numerous mechanisms for cell to cell contact.
   E. All of the above.

3) Epithelial tissues are generally:
   A. Composed of a dense population of cells.
   B. Active in mitosis throughout life.
   C. Avascular.
   D. Supported by an underlying connective tissue.
   E. All of the above.

4) Mucous membranes:
   A. Line closed cavities.
   B. Line cavities and canals which connect with the external environment.
   C. Invariably contain mucous glands.
   D. Never contain serous glands.
   E. Are avascular.

5) Epithelia in which all of the component cells rest on the basement membrane but not all reach the apical surface is termed:
   A. Simple squamous.
   B. Stratified.
   C. Pseudostratified.
   D. Endothelium.
   E. Urothelium.

6) An example of stratified secretory epithelium may be found in the:
A. Duodenum.
B. Walls of large lymphatic vessels.
C. Central canal of the spinal cord.
D. Endocervical glands.
E. Sebaceous glands.

7) The mode of secretion in which a small apical portion of the cytoplasm is lost during the secretory process is termed:
A. Holocrine.
B. Merocrine.
C. Eccrine.
D. Apocrine.
E. Endocrine.

8) Which of the following cells would be expected to exhibit zonulae occludentes (tight junctions)?
A. Neutrophilic leukocytes.
B. Simple columnar epithelial cells.
C. Osteoblasts.
D. Fat cells (lipocytes or adipocytes).
E. Macrophages.

9) Intracellular fibrils are well represented in all of the following EXCEPT:
A. Epithelial cells.
B. Connective tissue cells.
C. Cardiac muscle cells.
D. Skeletal muscle cells.
E. Nerve cells (neurons).

10) Which of the following cells is pluripotent and may differentiate into each of the other listed cells?
A. Endothelial cells.
B. Fibroblasts.
C. Fat cells.
D. Mesenchymal cells.
E. Chondroblasts.

11) The major component of the ground substance found in the adult connective tissues with generalized properties (connective tissue proper) is:
A. Tropocollagen.
B. Chondroitin sulfate.
C. Tropomyosin.
D. Hyaluronic acid.
E. Sialic acid.

12) Myoepithelial cells are:
   A. Found within the basal lamina of small vessels.
   B. Found within the basal lamina of some epithelia.
   C. Found within the basal lamina of skeletal myofibers.
   D. Arranged circumferentially about the ureter.
   E. None of the above.

13) Urothelium is unusual in that:
   A. It lacks a basement membrane.
   B. It secretes by the holocrine mode.
   C. Cellular junctions are lacking.
   D. Vascular elements are present within the epithelial component.
   E. The surface cells may be larger than those of lower levels and may occasionally be binucleate.

14) Wharton's jelly is an example of:
   A. Mucous connective tissue.
   B. Fibroadipose connective tissue.
   C. Pigmented connective tissue.
   D. Immature cartilaginous tissue.
   E. None of the above.

15) Which of the following is not a sulfated glycosaminoglycan?
   A. Dermatan sulfate.
   B. Chondroitin sulfate.
   C. Heparan sulfate.
   D. Keratan sulfate.
   E. Hyaluronic acid.

16) Which of following types of collagen fibers is associated with the basal lamina and lacks ultrastructural periodicity?
   A. Type I.
   B. Type II.
   C. Type III.
   D. Type IV.

17) Disregarding changes in diameter, the increase in the length of a long bone is effected by:
   A. Appositional growth of the epiphyseal cartilage only.
   B. Interstitial growth of the epiphyseal cartilage only.
   C. Appositional growth of boney tissue only.
   D. Appositional growth of boney tissue and interstitial growth of cartilage.
   E. Appositional growth of both cartilage and boney tissue.

18) The predominant type of collagen produced by the chondroblasts of the hyaline type of cartilaginous tissue is:
   A. Type I.
   B. Type II.
   C. Type III.
   D. Type IV.
   E. Type V.

19) Circulating blood cells which contain granules with antihistaminic activity include:
   A. Monocytes.
   B. Eosinophils.
   C. Basophils.
   D. Neutrophils.
   E. Mast cells.

20) Reticular fibers:
   A. Are easily visualized in routine tissue sections.
   B. Can not be visualized with silver impregnation methods.
   C. Are identical to actin microfilaments.
   D. Are chemically similar to Type I collagen fibers but lack periodicity.
   E. Are PAS positive and display 64 nm periodicity.

21) Each of the following cell types is capable of producing ground substance <u>EXCEPT</u>:
   A. Chondroblast.
   B. Fibroblast.
   C. Mesenchymal cell.
   D. Osteoblast.
   E. Erythroblast.

22) Fibroblasts are the predominate cell type present in:
   A. Reticular connective tissue.
   B. Adipose connective tissue.
   C. Mesenchyme.
   D. Dense regular connective tissue.
   E. Osseous tissue.

23) The <u>organic</u> component of bone is:
   A. Chondroitin sulfate.
   B. Elastin.
   C. Osteoid.
   D. Hydroxyapatite.
   E. None of the above.

24) A goblet cell:
   A. May be considered a unicellular gland.
   B. Possesses a well-developed Golgi apparatus.
   C. Secretes periodically instead of continuously.
   D. Contains secretory granules which stain poorly with eosin.
   E. All of the above.

25) The organelle that binds and releases calcium during relaxation and contraction of skeletal muscle is the:
   A. Golgi apparatus.
   B. Mitochondrion.
   C. Lysosome.
   D. Transverse (T) tubule.
   E. Sarcoplasmic reticulum.

26) The "triad" of skeletal muscle consists of:
   A. One "T" tubule bounded laterally by two terminal cisterns of the sarcoplasmic reticulum.
   B. Two "T" tubules bounded laterally by one terminal cistern of the sarcoplasmic reticulum.
   C. One "T" tubule bounded by one terminal cisterns of the sarcoplasmic reticulum.
   D. Two "T" tubules bounded by two fenestrated cisterns of the sarcoplasmic reticulum.
   E. None of the above.

27) Intercalated discs in cardiac muscle are always located at the position of the:
   A. Junction of the A and I bands.
   B. Z disc.
   C. M line.
   D. Motor end plate.
   E. None of the above.

28) In normal contraction of the sarcomere:
   A. Only the A band shortens.
   B. Only the I band shortens.
   C. Both the A and I bands shorten.
   D. Both the A and H bands shorten.
   E. Both the I and H bands shorten.

29) The specific cytoplasmic granules of granulocytes are apparent within which stage of differentiation?
   A. CFU cell.
   B. Myeloblast.
   C. Promyelocyte.
   D. Myelocyte.
   E. None of the above.

30) Primary granules of granular leukocytes:
   A. Form after the secondary (specific) granules.
   B. Are largely lysosomal in nature.
   C. Both A and B are correct.
   D. Neither A nor B is correct.

31) Gemmules are:
   A. Axoaxonic synapses.
   B. Axonic spines.
   C. Axodendritic synapses.
   D. Dendritic spines.
   E. Axosomatic synapses.

32) Most nerve cells (neurons) are:
   A. Bipolar.
   B. Unipolar.
   C. Multipolar.
   D. Spindle-shaped.
   E. Spherical.

33) Astrocytes may perform all of the following functions within the nervous tissue EXCEPT:
   A. Formation of perivascular end feet (sucker feet).
   B. Formation of myelin.
   C. Participation in the transport of metabolites between neurons and blood.
   D. Reaction to injury and repair of damaged neuropil.
   E. Support of both gray and white matter within the brain and spinal cord.

34) The cytoplasm within the axon is often referred to as the:
   A. Axoplasm.
   B. Neurolemma.
   C. Axolemma.
   D. Neuropil.
   E. Perikaryon.

35) Which of the following statements is correct concerning smooth muscle?
   A. Motor end plates are present between each muscle cell and a lower motor neuron.
   B. The "T" tubules are much smaller than those of skeletal and cardiac muscle and occur with terminal cisterns of sarcoplasmic reticulum both as "diads" and "triads".
   C. Neither actin nor myosin filaments are present within the cell.
   D. Contraction can be elicited by neural, hormonal and myotactic (stretch) mechanisms.
   E. The intercalated disks occur only at the A-I junctions.

**CHANGE IN FORMAT:** For each of the following questions select:

(A) if only 1, 2 and 3 are correct.
(B) if only 1 and 3 are correct.
(C) if only 2 and 4 are correct.
(D) if only 4 is correct.
(E) if all are correct.

36) Which of the following connective tissue cells can be identified easily and with a high degree of confidence in routine hematoxylin and eosin preparations of areolar connective tissue?
1. Eosinophils.
2. Plasma cells.
3. Fat cells.
4. Mast cells.

37) Nissl substance or bodies are:
1. Aggregated, flattened cisternae of rough endoplasmic reticulum with numerous free ribosomes at the electron microscopic level.
2. Basophilic clumps at the light microscopic level.
3. Absent from the axon hillock of the neuron.
4. Found in only medium- to large-sized multipolar neurons.

38) Which cells may be involved in the formation of myelin?
1. Microglia.
2. Schwann cells.
3. Fibrous astrocytes.
4. Oligodendroglia.

39) A Haversian system or osteon consists of:
1. Osteocytes and concentric lamellae.
2. Haversian canals and interstitial lamellae.
3. Haversian canals.
4. Outer and inner circumferential lamellae.

40) The "T" or transverse tubules of muscle are:
1. Continuous with the sarcolemma.
2. Part of the smooth endoplasmic reticulum.
3. A characteristic feature of cardiac and skeletal muscle.
4. Part of the rough endoplasmic reticulum.

41) A sarcomere is:
1. The smallest repeating unit of the myofibril in skeletal and cardiac muscle.
2. Composed of one complete A band and one-half of two adjoining I bands.
3. Delimited on both ends by a Z disc.
4. The term applied to muscle mitochondria.

**(A) = 1, 2, 3 (B) = 1, 3 (C) = 2, 4 (D) = 4 only (E) = All**

42) The Purkinje cells of cardiac muscle:
   1. Are larger in average size than regular cardiac muscle cells.
   2. Stain more lightly that regular cardiac muscle cells.
   3. Are modified to conduct the impulse for contraction.
   4. Contain more contractile filaments than regular cardiac muscle cells.

43) Osteoclasts:
   1. Resorb bony tissue.
   2. Synthesize osteoid.
   3. Secrete hydrolytic (lysosomal) enzymes.
   4. May differentiate into osteoblasts if the need arises.

44) Retention of Schwann cell cytoplasm within the myelin lamellae results in the presence of curious structures known as:
   1. Nodes of Ranvier.
   2. Neurokeratin.
   3. Internodes.
   4. Schmidt-Lanterman incisures.

45) The cell bodies of spinal, cranial and autonomic ganglia are surrounded or encapsulated by:
   1. Oligodendroglial cells.
   2. Astroblasts.
   3. Reticulum cells.
   4. Satellite cells.

46) Eosinophilic leukocytes:
   1. Become phagocytic in the presence of antigen-antibody complexes.
   2. Exhibit ameboid movement.
   3. May be present in increased numbers during parasitic infestation or in allergic states.
   4. Possess specific granules which contain histamine.

47) The secretory portion of simple glands may be:
   1. Straight.
   2. Coiled.
   3. Branched tubular.
   4. Branched alveolar.

**(A) = 1, 2, 3 (B) = 1, 3 (C) = 2, 4 (D) = 4 only (E) = All**

48) Microglia are:
 1. Developmentally related to blood monocytes.
 2. Mesodermal in origin.
 3. Phagocytic.
 4. Found both within the central nervous system and the peripheral nervous system.

49) Neurons in the central nervous system:
 1. Are all similar in size.
 2. Divide mitotically.
 3. Possess only chemical synapses.
 4. In certain locations may contain neuromelanin pigment.

50) Ependymal cells:
 1. Line the brain ventricles and central canal of the spinal cord.
 2. May possess surface cilia in some point of their vital period.
 3. Are joined to each other with tight junctions.
 4. Represent the apical cells of the neural tube epithelium and may possess basal processes which ramify into the neural parenchyma to end on blood vessels.

# UNIT III: ORGANS AND SYSTEMS

Organs consist of an orderly arrangement of tissues in such a form that they work together in unison to enable the organ to perform its specialized function. More simplistically, organs are, for the most part, discrete anatomic and functional units. Most organs are composed of several tissue types. Usually, a single tissue is of major functional importance and the other tissues provide structural and physiologic support. The primary tissue of an organ is referred to as the parenchyma . An organ's parenchymal component comprises one of the four basic tissue types: epithelia, connective tissue, muscular tissue or nervous tissue. The supportive elements also consist of the same classes of tissues and within a single organ are collectively termed the stroma. In most cases, the parenchymal and stromal tissues are of different types. For instance, in a major salivary gland, like the parotid, the secretory and ductal epithelium which produce the serous product and transport it to the oral cavity constitute the parenchyma. The other tissues which enclose and intermingle with the parenchyma are the stroma. In this example, the stroma includes both the connective tissue that forms the capsule and that which supports the epithelial component within the gland (subepithelial connective tissue). The intrinsic vascular and nervous elements necessary for the function of the gland are also considered stromal elements.

The parenchymal and stromal components of most organs are arranged in one of two general patterns. If an organ is disposed around a lumen or cavity then it is considered a tubular or hollow organ. If the tissues that make up an organ are present in a more anatomically localized and solid form then the organ is regarded as a compact organ.

In tubular organs, the component tissues are arranged in concentric layers about the lumen or cavity in a specific manner. The tissue that interfaces directly with the luminal space or cavity is by definition an epithelium and comprises the parenchyma. The stroma consists of various alternating layers of muscular and connective tissue in which stromal vascular and nervous elements may be found. Depending on anatomic location, an additional epithelial layer may be present on the external surface of the organ (i.e. mesothelium) which may be referred to as the serosa. The serosa represents an additional stromal constituent. Many of the tubular organs are not delimited precisely from each other but are present as successive segments along the course of the luminal cavity. Tubular organs are distinguished by their regional differences in function and the often subtle structural modifications associated with their specific functional role. Examples of tubular organs include those forming certain segments of the digestive tract, respiratory passages, genitourinary tract and blood and lymphatic vascular channels.

Compact organs possess an extensive connective tissue framework, the stroma, that encloses and supports the parenchyma. The outermost connective tissue investment is called the capsule which defines the outer limits of the organ and is responsible for its anatomic localization at the macroscopic level. As a result, most compact organs can easily be dissected out and described as individual units. From the capsule, additional strands of connective tissue, termed trabeculae or septae, extend into the organ dividing it into compartments. Compartmentalization may be complete or incomplete. Often an indentation is evident on the capsular surface. This region is termed the hilus and serves as the point for the entry or exit of various vascular and nervous elements which contribute internally to the stroma. Usually a single artery enters at the hilus. Its major branches are found within the trabeculae or septae and the small terminal arteries extend into the parenchymal compartment where they give off capillaries. Veins and nerves follow the pattern of the arteries. Compact organs suspended within body cavities may also be covered externally by a serosa.

The parenchyma of compact organs is arranged in masses, cords, follicles, tubules, ducts or strands. In the kidney, for example, the parenchyma consists largely of the tubules of the nephron and the ducts which collect and transport the excretory product. In the thyroid, the parenchyma consists of epithelially-lined follicles filled with colloid and in the liver the epithelial cells of the parenchyma are present in a pattern of radiating cords. In some compact organs, the arrangement of the parenchyma is more or less consistent throughout the organ but in others separate functional regions with variations in structure may be present. Thus an external cortex and a deeper medulla may distinguished.

The human body contains over a hundred different organs. Most of these can be grouped into a much smaller number of organ systems. The individual organs that comprise an organ system collaborate to achieve the primary function of the particular system to which they belong. Thus all organs of a single organ system are specialized to carry out a related functional role and as such are structurally related as well. The study of the numerous organs of the body is simplified by viewing them as functional complexes known as systems. Each organ within a given system will, with few exceptions, be organized into either a tubular or compact pattern. If both the structural and functional relationships of the organs within an organ system are appreciated and the basic pattern of structural arrangement for each organ is considered, then only the exceptions to these generalized concepts and the functionally-related structural modifications of the parenchymal cells need be recalled.

# THE NERVOUS SYSTEM

It is appropriate to make the transition from the study of tissues to consideration of the organs which comprise the various systems by way of the nervous system. This is because the parenchyma of all the nervous organs (nervous tissue) is visually prominent and compositionally predominate. Conversely, the stromal elements (vessels and connective tissue) are largely inconspicuous and contribute little to total organ mass. Nonetheless, the importance of stroma as a structural component of a nervous organ is paramount. Without the presence of the stromal elements and their functional interaction with nervous tissue, the organ would be unable to function in its specialized role.

The organs of the central nervous system include the cerebrum, cerebellum, choroid plexi and spinal cord. Principal organs of the peripheral nervous system include the peripheral nerves and the various ganglia. The ganglia are classified by their functions and can be distinguished by certain morphologic characteristics in tissue sections. Specifically represented in the PNS are sensory ganglia (dorsal root and cranial) and motor ganglia of both sympathetic and parasympathetic limbs of the autonomic nervous system.

## Organs of the Central Nervous System

The major organs of the CNS (cerebrum, cerebellum and spinal cord) are all structurally and functionally interconnected. Because of their functional importance in the continued viability of their owner and their susceptibility to damage by even slight direct physical trauma, they are enclosed and protected by bones. As an added protective measure, they are invested by special coverings (meninges) and a layer of liquid, the cerebral spinal fluid (CSF). The CSF is produced by another CNS organ, the choroid plexus.

### External Investments

The meninges cover the outer surfaces of the cerebrum, cerebellum and spinal cord. The outermost layer is termed the dura mater or pachymeninx and consists of dense fibrous connective tissue. The dura mater which encloses the brain and that of the spinal cord differ.

Cerebral dura serves as a protective covering for the brain and also as the fibrous periosteum of certain cranial bones. In addition to its connective tissue component, the periosteal aspect contains many blood vessels and nerves.

The spinal dura consists of a single layer of dense fibrous connective tissue. The vertebrae which enclose the cord are covered separately by periosteum. Between the periosteum and spinal dura lies the epidural space. In the spinal cord this is a true space and contains many thin-walled veins that anastomose freely and lie within a loose connective tissue that contains many fat cells (adipose tissue). Exiting spinal nerves traverse the epidural space. Injection of anesthetic agents into this space is sometimes performed to effect an "epidural block".

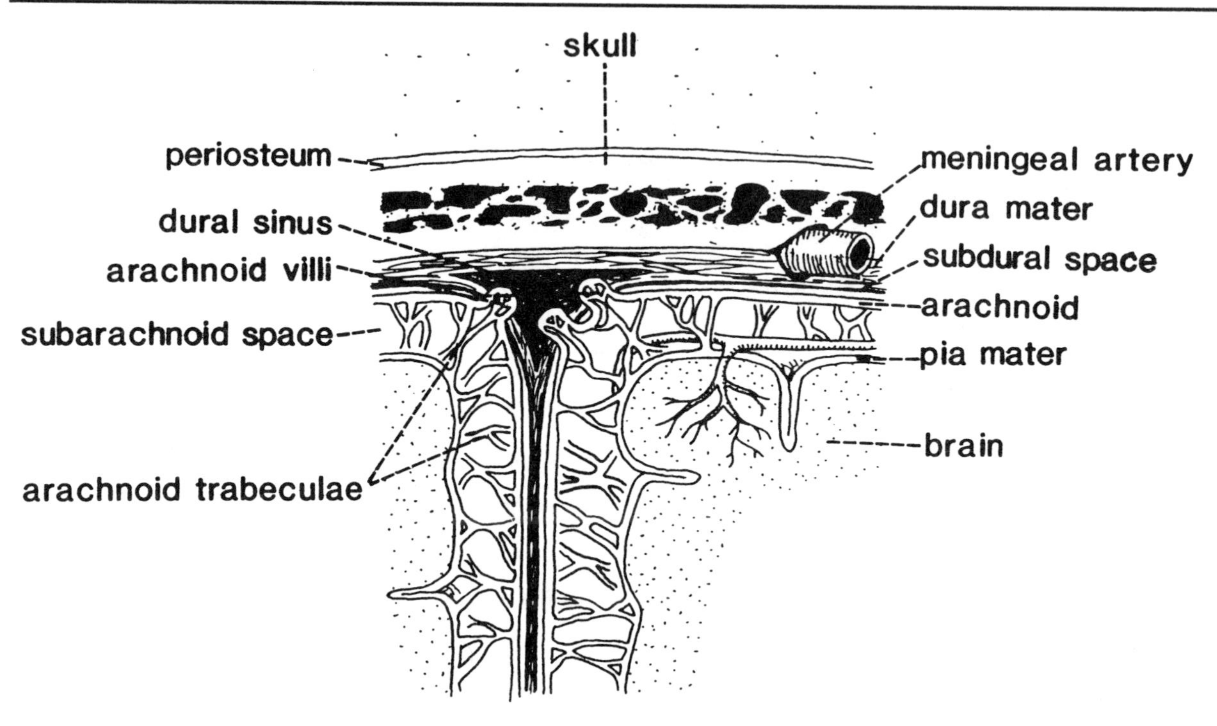


**Fig. 3.1.** Relationships of the cerebral meninges.

The inner layers of the meninges are the arachnoid and pia mater which collectively comprise the leptomeninges. Between the outermost layer of the leptomeninges, the arachnoid, and the dura of both brain and spinal cord is a narrow subdural space containing a lymph-like fluid.

The arachnoid is a thin, delicate and avascular membrane that lines the dura mater. It passes over the surface of the brain without entering the depths of the convolutions. Thin cord-like trabeculae pass from the arachnoid to the pia mater. A substantial space is present between the closely apposed arachnoid membrane and the pia mater, the so-called subarachnoid space. The space is traversed by the arachnoidal trabeculae and is filled with the cerebral spinal fluid produced by the choroid plexi. The arachnoidal trabeculae of the brain are more numerous than those of the spinal cord.

The innermost layer of the leptomeninges is the pia mater. It closely invests both the brain and spinal cord and extends into the depths of the cerebral sulci and extends into the anterior median fissure of the cord. The more superficial layer of the pia, often referred to as epipial tissue, is composed of a network of collagenous fibers closely apposed to the overlying arachnoid. The deeper, inner layer, called the intima pia, contains elastic and reticular fibers. Within the pia are the blood vessels that serve the underlying neural tissue. As blood vessels pass into neural tissue they take with them a covering of intima pia. In the case of larger vessels, an intervening perivascular space continuous with the subarachnoid space is present.

## Arachnoid Villi

In some areas of the brain, the arachnoid penetrates the dura mater to form so-called arachnoid villi. These structures lie within the venous sinuses formed by the dura and are particularly prominent on either side of the midsagittal fissure on the surface of the cerebrum in association with the superior sagittal sinus. The arachnoid villi function in the vascular resorption of CSF.

## Structure of the Cerebrum

In the cerebral hemispheres, gray matter is located on the surface of the brain as the cerebral cortex and deep or centrally, surrounded by white matter, as ganglia or nuclei. The surface of the cerebral hemispheres is convoluted which significantly increases its surface area and thus the amount of cortical gray matter. Surface projections of folds are termed gyri while the intervening depressions are called sulci. The cerebral cortex is continuous along all the convolutions and fissures. The phylogenetically older and less complex hippocampus and olfactory cortex is referred to as the allocortex. The rest, which comprises the majority of the cerebral cortex, is termed the isocortex. The cortex contains neurons, fibers (axons, dendrites), neuroglia and blood vessels. The neurons are often classified by shape and include:

1) Pyramidal cells
2) Stellate (granule) cells
3) Fusiform (horizontal) cells
4) Inverted (Martinotti) cells

The cells of the cerebral cortex tend to be arranged in horizontal layers or lamina. Homotypic areas of the isocortex are characterized by the presence of six layers. In heterotypic areas and the allocortex, alteration of the six basic layers may occur. The named layers of the typical isocortex include:

1) <u>Molecular layer</u> composed mainly of fibers from cells in the deeper layers which tend to run parallel to the surface of the cerebrum and a few neurons, the horizon-

tal cells (of Cajal).

2) <u>External granular layer</u> contains small, triangular nerve cell bodies.
3) <u>External pyramidal layer</u> consists of large pyramidal cells and many small stellate cells.
4) <u>Internal granular layer</u> contains many small stellate or granule cells.
5) <u>Internal pyramidal (ganglionic) layer</u> composed mostly of large- and medium-sized pyramidal cells.
6) <u>Multiform of polymorphic cell layer</u> contains cells of varying size and shape. Also present are the inverted cells (of Martinotti) which are pyramidal in shape but possess axons that, unlike other cortical neurons, extend toward the surface of the cerebrum.

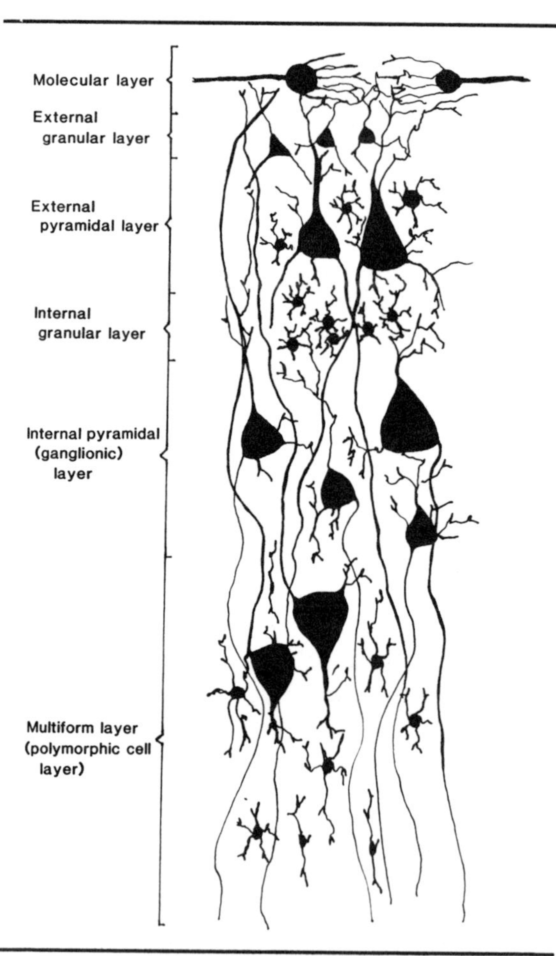


**Fig. 3.2.** Layers of the cerebral isocortex.

It should be noted that all the layers contain fibers, neuroglial cells and vascular elements as well as the neuronal populations just described.

The white matter lies below the cortex and surrounds the central areas of gray matter which also contain neurons. White matter is composed of bundles of myelinated and unmyelinated fibers passing in all directions. Depending on the origin and destination of the fiber bundles (tracts) they are classified as:

1) Association fibers connect different parts of the cerebral cortex within the same hemisphere.
2) Commissural fibers connect cortical regions in different hemispheres.
3) Projection fibers connect the cortex with lower centers.

## Structure of the Cerebellum

The cerebellum consists of right and left hemispheres connected by a median lobe, the vermis. Transverse fissures divide the cerebellum into lobules. On the surface are numerous folds or folia. Gray matter is located on the surface as a thin cortex overlying the centrally located white matter. The white matter surrounds additional gray matter, the cerebellar nuclei.

The cerebellar cortex consists of three microscopically prominent layers:

1) The outer molecular layer contains a few small neurons and many nonmyelinated fibers.
2) The middle layer is occupied by a single row of large neurons (Purkinje cells) and is termed the Purkinje cell layer.
3) The innermost layer of numerous small neurons or granule cells is called the granular cell layer. It also contains a few so-called Golgi neurons.

The neurons of the granular cell layer are small, contain 3 to 6 dendrites and a nonmyelinated axon that ascends to the molecular layer where it divides into two lateral branches that run along the length of the folium. The Purkinje cells are large, flask-shaped cells with a profusely branched dendrite which is located within the molecular layer. The arborized dendrite fans out within a single plane which is oriented at a right angle to the long axis of the folium and to the lateral branches of granular cell axonal processes. Basket cells are located within the region of the Purkinje cells. These small neurons send out axonal processes which make multiple contacts with the soma and initial axonal segments of several Purkinje cells. The axons of the Purkinje cells traverse the granular cell layer to synapse with cells in the cerebellar nuclei. The axons may also send off ascending collaterals which may enter other parts of the cerebellar cortex. In the cortex are also found the terminations of mossy and climbing fibers. The climbing fibers are largely recurrent axonal collaterals from neurons of the cerebellar nuclei. They ascend unbranched into the molecular layer where they run parallel to and synapse with the dendritic trees of the Purkinje cells. The mossy fibers originate outside the cerebellum. These axons are often highly branched and usually a single branch will terminate on one of the dendrites of a granule cell in the granular cell layer.

CEREBELLAR CORTEX

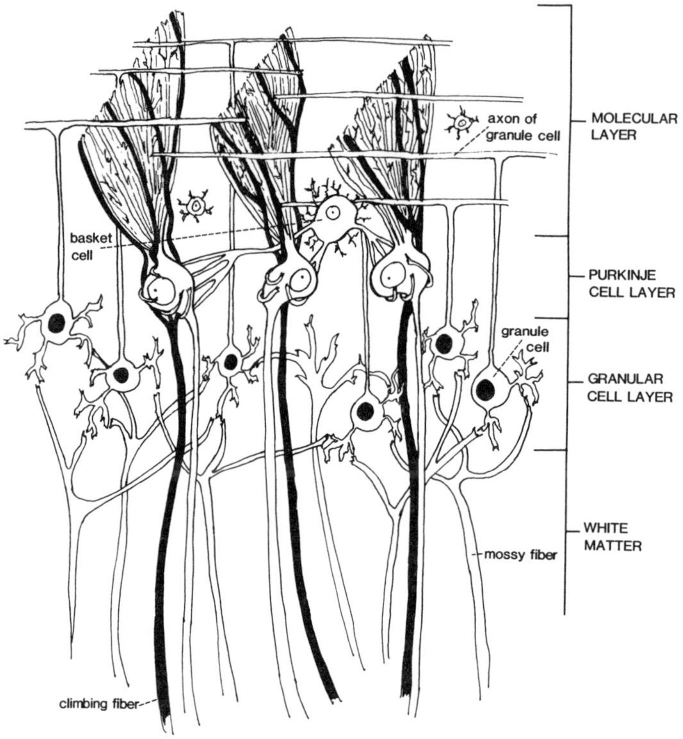

**Fig. 3.3.** Layers of the cerebellar cortex.

## Structure of the Spinal Cord

The cord is roughly oval in shape and varies in shape and structure at different levels. Posteriorly, it is divided into left and right halves by the dorsal median septum. Anteriorly, it is divided into halves by the ventral median fissure. The entire cord is invested by the meninges. The pia mater fails to enter the dorsal median septum but extends into the ventral median fissure. The central portion of the cord consists of gray matter disposed in a "butterfly" pattern. In a cross-section the gray matter is divided into anterior horns and posterior horns at the position of the central canal. The somatic efferent motor neurons (lower motor neurons) are located in the anterior horns. They are especially numerous in the cervical and lumbar enlargements which are associated with the upper and lower limb musculature, respectively. Their axons contribute to the motor branches of the brachial and lumbar plexi. The central canal, lined by ependyma, is located within the center of the gray matter. At the site of entrance of the dorsal root fibers on both sides, a shallow dorsal lateral sulcus is present. White matter is peripherally disposed about the gray matter and is divided into longitudinal columns or funiculi. The dorsal funiculus lies between the dorsal median septum and the dorsal horn. The remaining white matter comprises the ventrolateral funiculus. It may be subdivided by the position of the ventral horn and incoming ventral nerve roots into a lateral funiculus which lies between the two gray horns and a ventral funiculus which lies between the ventral horn and the ventral median fissure.

### Choroid Plexus

The choroid plexi are located in all four of the brain ventricles. They are composed of complex folds and invaginations of telae choroideae which consists of a modified layer of ependymal cells and an underlying highly vascularized pia mater. The ependymal lining is simple cuboidal to low columnar. By electron microscopy irregular, bulbous microvilli are observed and basally located occluding (tight) junctions are present. The capillaries within the pial component are unlike other CNS capillaries in that they are fenestrated. The function of the choroid plexus is to secrete the CSF.

## Organs of the Peripheral Nervous System

The peripheral nerves course throughout the body and when associated with specific connective tissue and vascular elements comprise small intrinsic organs within various named organs and body parts. Small collections of neurons are also found within the body outside the CNS. These PNS organs are termed ganglia.

### Peripheral Nerves

The investment of PNS neurites by Schwann cells and the process of myelination and myelin structure have already been discussed. Groups of nerve fibers, both myelinated and nonmyelinated are often bundled together, reinforced and metabolically supported by connective tissues into peripheral nerve trunks. Enclosing an entire nerve trunk is the epineurium, a thick fibrous sheath of connective tissue which contains blood vessels and adipocytes. The epineurium may extend into the nerve to separate it into several nerve fascicles. The individual fascicles are further ensheathed by the perineurium. The innermost connective tissue investment is a thin, delicate layer of reticular fibers known as the endoneurium which surrounds the individual axons within the fascicles.

## Peripheral Ganglia

The peripheral ganglia are collections of neurons located outside the CNS. They vary in size from those containing only a few nerve cells to those in which as many as 50,000 or more neurons may be found. The ganglia, like peripheral nerve trunks, are covered externally by connective tissue investments. They can be grouped into craniospinal (sensory) and autonomic (motor).

1) Craniospinal ganglia - sensory, and include the dorsal root ganglia (spinal) and similar swellings along some cranial nerves (V, VII, IX, X). Neurons are unipolar and are surrounded by satellite cells. The neurons tend to be collected into small groups and their nuclei are centrally located. For the most part, synapses are absent.
2) Autonomic ganglia - motor, and include both sympathetic (chain and collateral) and parasympathetic (located near or within the organs that they serve). The neurons are multipolar and send out a single, nonmyelinated axon (post-ganglionic visceral efferent). The neurons tend to be smaller than the sensory ganglion cells, do not appear in groups and often contain eccentrically placed nuclei. They are surrounded by satellite cells. Synapses occur within the ganglia (preganglionic axons synapse on the ganglion cells).

## IMMUNE SYSTEM

### Components of the Immune System

The functional cells of the immune system are the phagocytes and lymphocytes. Phagocytes are present in the circulating blood and connective tissues as neutrophils and widely distributed throughout the body as elements of the monocyte/macrophage system. Many other cells are capable of modulating and participating in immune-related events such as eosinophils, basophils and mast cells. Lymphocytes are not phagocytic but play an important part in immune competency and modulation of immune reactions. They are found within the reticular connective tissue of the bone marrow, as one of the cellular elements in the circulating blood, as one component of the migratory cell population of the connective tissues and as the major parenchymal component of the lymphoid organs. These include the lymph nodes, tonsils, thymus and spleen.

### Lymphocytes

There are two major types, depending on whether they are subjected to the influence of the thymus during development or not. The thymic-derived population is referred to as T-cells or T-lymphocytes. The other population develops independent of thymic influence, probably in the bone marrow and the cells are called B-cells or B-lymphocytes. These two cell types are morphologically indistinguishable but functionally distinct. T-lymphocytes are important in cell-mediated immunity whereas their B-cell counterparts function in humoral immune responses. Specialized methods for their differentiation have been devised.

#### B-Lymphocyte Identification

1) B-cells possess surface immunoglobulin (sIg) which is specific for the antigen the cell has been preprogrammed to recognize.

2) B-cells form rosettes with sheep erythrocytes that have been treated with immunoglobulin (IgM) and complement, ($C_3$) termed EAC-rosettes.

3) B-cells have unique surface antigens (markers) present on the outer surface of their plasma membranes.

#### T-Lymphocyte Identification

1) T-cells rosette naturally with untreated sheep erythrocytes, so-called E-rosettes.

2) T-cells also have unique surface antigens that can be demonstrated with special immunocytologic techniques. Subpopulations of T-cells may also be defined in this manner (i.e., helper T-cells and suppressor T-cells).

## Generation and Differentiation of Lymphocytes

The progenitors of B-lymphocytes arise directly from the bone marrow whereas T-lymphocyte progenitors leave the bone marrow to reside in the thymus. During the generation of each type of progenitor, it acquires the capacity to recognize a single antigen. T- and B-cell progenitors each capable of recognizing one of more than 30,000 different antigens are produced. Curiously, this programming process occurs in the absence of antigen. Once the antigen specificity is acquired by either a pre-T- or pre-B-cell it remains fixed for each individual cell and all of its progeny.

Pre-T-cells that leave the bone marrow are incompetent to mount an immune response and must reside in the thymus in order to complete a second phase in their maturation. When they leave the thymus as small lymphocytes (post-T-cells) they are still functionally immature. Once they encounter their antigen, if ever, they become activated and undergo blastic transformation to produce a variety of effector T-cells each with the same unique antigen specificity as the progenitor. These effector cells comprise the so-called functional subsets of T-cells. Included are cytotoxic T-cells (killer T-cells) which are capable of direct killing of foreign cells, helper T-cells and suppressor T-cells both which modulate B-cell function.

Pre-B-cells develop functional maturity sometime after leaving the bone marrow and without the influence of the thymus. When they leave, they take up residence in various locations. The most important of these are the lymphoid organs because they are located so that there is maximal exposure to antigens in the blood (spleen) and in the lymph (lymph nodes). They also reside in areas close to the external environment (tonsils, Peyer's patches of gut, diffuse lymphoid tissue below epithelia). Once they encounter their specific antigen they undergo morphologic changes (blastic transformation) and proliferate to produce many more B-cells with identical antigen specificity. Many of the progeny differentiate into the effector cells of humoral immunity, the terminally differentiated plasma cells, while others remain in the proliferative pool. When antigen is no longer present, proliferation ceases but the plasma cells already produced live and contribute antibody for several days or weeks afterward. Cells in the proliferative pool do not continue to differentiate into plasma cells in the absence of antigen but instead are converted into memory B-cells that live for several years. Their presence allows a more rapid response of greater intensity upon a second encounter with the same antigen (anamnestic response).

## Lymphoid Tissue

This term does not refer to a specific type of tissue but rather to aggregates of lymphocytes in connective tissues usually below epithelia. The collections of lymphocytes may be present as diffuse aggregates, so-called diffuse lymphoid tissue, or in the form of more localized structures known as lymphoid nodules. These consist of a dense spherical collection of lymphocytes characterized by the presence of a light staining central region, the germinal center, composed chiefly of lymphoblasts, which in turn is surrounded by a dense aggregate of small, darkly stained lymphocytes. Lymph nodules indicate antigen stimulation and B-cell proliferation and are transitory structures. Similar structures are present in certain of the lymphoid organs.

## Thymus

The thymus is a bi-lobed, encapsulated lymphoid organ found in the anterior mediastinum. Unlike other lymphoid organs that are predominately reticular connective tissue, the thymus possesses an epithelial reticulum derived from the endoderm of the third and perhaps the fourth pharyngeal pouches. The subsequent infiltration of large numbers of lymphocytes into the epithelium probably induces blood vessels to grow in to nourish them. It is unusual for an epithelium to contain blood vessels as epithelia are usually avascular. The epithelial component is present in a three-dimensional network (reticulum) but does not produce fibers. The epithelial reticulum provides a suitable microenvironment for the proliferation and maturational sequence of developing T-lymphocytes and constitutes an important component of the blood-thymic barrier that protects the developing T-cells from blood-borne antigens. Correspondingly, no lymph-borne antigens enter the thymus due to absence of afferent lymphatics.

The two lobes of the thymus are divided into lobules by septa. The septa are thin connective tissue components which contain blood vessels supplying the thymus. All lobules have a cortex and a medulla. The cortex is the outer zone containing dense aggregates of lymphocytes which are arranged diffusely. Lymphoid nodules are not present because they are a characteristic of B-cells and the thymus contains T-cells. All cortices are separated from each other by the septa. The medulla is the underlying pale staining zone which is continuous from one lobule to the next. Located within the thymic medulla are curious structures known as Hassall's corpuscles. These small eosinophilic whorls represent concentric layers of flat epithelial cells that tend to keratinize. Their presence is virtually diagnostic for thymus.

## Lymph Nodes

Lymph nodes are bean-shaped lymphoid organs interposed along the course of larger lymphatic vessels. Individually, they are covered over most of their surface by a capsule which is interrupted on the concave surface by the presence of a hilus. At this site, arteries and veins enter and leave, respectively. Nerves are also present as is an efferent lymphatic vessel. Afferent lymphatic vessels, usually many, enter the lymph node on its convex surface. The capsule extends into the substance of the node as trabeculae. The substance of the node consists of an outer cortex and inner medulla. Lymph nodes are composed of reticular connective tissue in which large aggregates of lymphocytes are present. They constantly filter the lymph to detect lymph-borne antigenic substances and when encountered become a site of immune-reactivity.

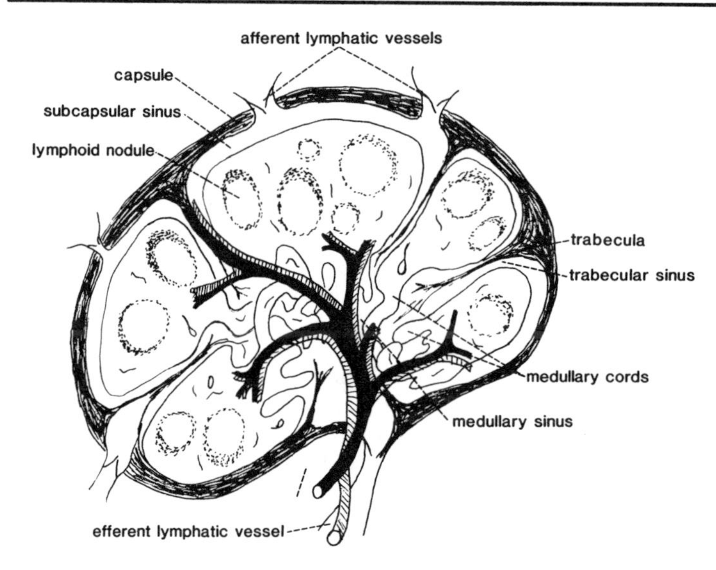


**Fig. 3.4.** Structure of a lymph node.

The cortex contains many lymphoid nodules (follicles). Depending on the state of antigenic stimulation, the nodules may contain germinal (follicular) centers. Between the nodules is an area referred to as the paracortical or parafollicular zone, it is a T-cell area. The cortical tissue extends downward as finger-like projections into the medulla as medullary cords.

The medulla stains lighter with routine stains as fewer cells reside there. The cells present consist of lymphocytes, plasma cells, macrophages and reticulum cells. The medulla is traversed by many lymph vascular spaces termed medullary sinuses. These are lined by endothelial cells that possess frequent intercellular gaps. Other sinuses are present and are interconnected. Just below the capsule is a narrow subcapsular sinus. It is connected with the trabecular sinuses which follow along the trabeculae. Trabecular sinuses are confluent with the paracortical sinuses which drain into the medullary sinuses. These structures allow the continuous flow of lymph through the node so that its immune-competent cell collection can react to antigens brought in from local tissues drained by the nodes. Lymph flows in through many afferent vessels to enter the subcapsular sinus. It then is able to enter the cortex along the trabeculae within the trabecular sinuses. The lymph leaves the cortex via the paracortical sinuses which drain into the medulla through the medullary sinuses. The medullary sinuses are confluent with an efferent lymphatic vessel.

The circulation of lymphocytes between tissue and lymph nodes is an important part of immune activity. Curiously, there are very few lymphocytes in the afferent lymph, many more are present in the efferent lymph. Some of the exiting lymphocytes are produced in the node while the majority (recirculating lymphocytes) have entered the node via the blood vascular system. Lymphocytes circulating in the blood enter the node by way of peculiar post-capillary venules located in the paracortical areas. These venules are lined by cuboidal endothelial cells and it is possible that they possess surface receptors that are recognized by the lymphocytes.

## Spleen

During fetal life the spleen serves as a hematopoietic organ and it retains the capacity to produce blood cells throughout life if the need arises. The major role of the spleen is to filter blood. Unlike lymph nodes, it does not filter lymph and therefore does not possess afferent lymphatics. The spleen is enclosed in a thick, dense fibrous tissues capsule. Connective tissue trabeculae extend from the capsule into the substance of the organ. The trabeculae contain the larger blood vessels which are continuous with the splenic artery and vein entering and exiting at the splenic hilus, respectively. The main substance of the spleen is a soft material known as the splenic pulp. Splenic pulp consists of white pulp and red pulp.

### White Pulp

The white pulp is represented by spherical aggregates of lymphoid tissue. They may be seen grossly and are termed Malpighian corpuscles. These lymphoid masses are found in association with a central artery which they surround. The central artery is actually an arteriole and most often is located in an eccentric position within the lymphoid tissue that envelopes it. As arteries (arterioles) leave the trabeculae they become ensheathed with lymphoid tissue, the so-called periarteriolar lymphoid sheath (PALS). At various points along the course of these vessels, the lymphoid tissue increases in amount to form the splenic nodules. The PALS is a T-cell zone. Lymphoid nodules replete with germinal centers may appear at the periphery of the PALS. The nodules represent areas of B-cell proliferation. The PALS represents collections of recirculating T-cells which enter the spleen at the interface of the white pulp with the red pulp, the so-called marginal zone.

## Red Pulp

With the exception of the connective tissue of the capsule and trabeculae and the white pulp, all else is termed red pulp. The red pulp is an area where the blood is filtered and exposed to immune-related cells such as macrophages. It contains many venous sinuses which are perhaps the terminal ramifications of the central arteriole on the venous side of the circulation. The walls of the venous sinuses are unusual in that they have slit-like spaces between the elongate and longitudinally disposed endothelial cells (rod or littoral cells). They lack typical intercellular junctions but are enclosed by a highly fenestrated basement membrane. Between two adjacent venous sinuses is an intervening pulp cord (cord of Billroth). The cords of Billroth are continuous with the PALS. The arrangement of pulp sinuses and cords is the basis for the filtration system of the spleen and enables it to remove senescent blood cells and circulating particulate material including microorganisms. The spleen is also the site of production of a large amount of the circulating antibody by mature plasma cells.

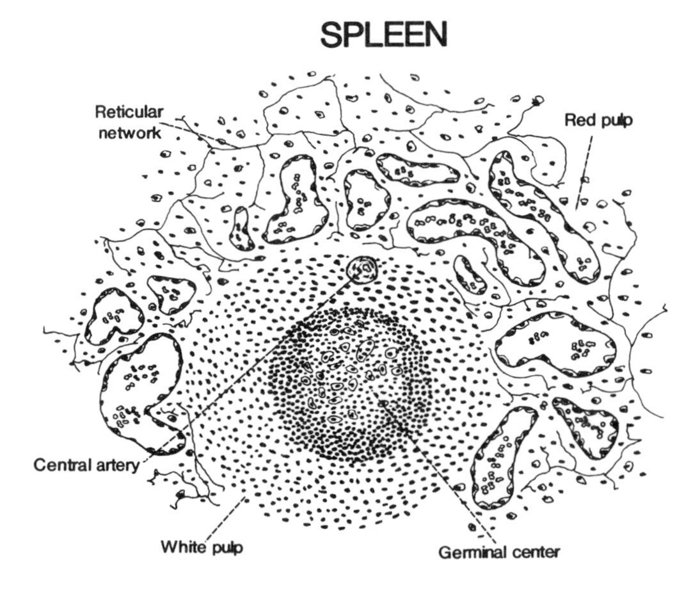


**Fig. 3.5.** Splenic red and white pulp.

## Blood Flow in the Spleen

Blood enters the spleen in the splenic artery which branches and follows the trabeculae as trabecular arteries which then leave the trabeculae as the central arterioles. Progressively, these become smaller with many parallel branches, the penicillar arteries (arteries of the red pulp). Each penicilli then branches into two to three capillaries with thick walls, the so-called sheathed capillaries (Schweigger-Seidel sheath). The sheathed capillaries eventually continue as simple capillaries. The termination of these capillaries is controversial. Two theories attempt to explain how the terminal capillaries connect with the venous sinuses to complete the circulation of blood through the spleen. In the open or slow circulation model, the terminal arterial capillaries open directly into the pulp reticulum and the blood slowly filters back into venous sinuses. In the closed or rapid circulation model, the terminal arterial capillaries open directly into the venous sinuses. It is possible that both methods operate in the human spleen.

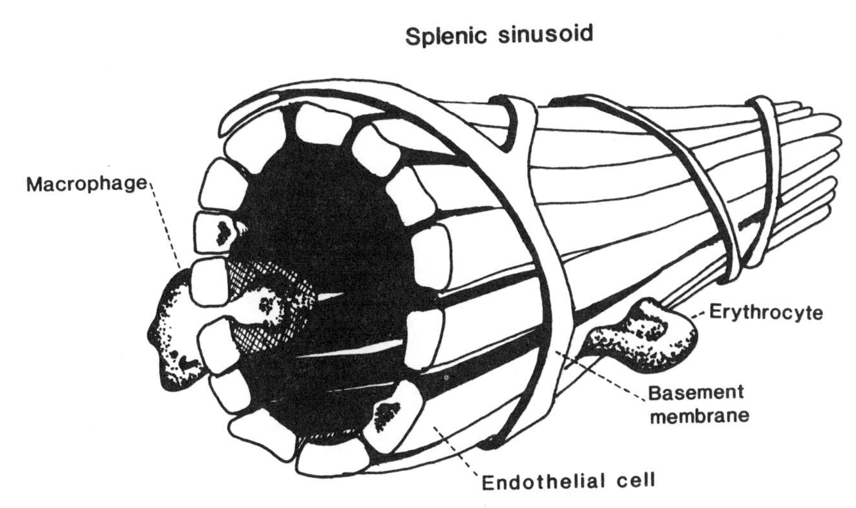


**Fig. 3.6.** Structure of the splenic sinusoid.

## Tonsils

The tonsils represent dense collections of lymphocytes associated with reticular connective tissue and are located below a surfacing epithelium. They are considered organs because they are discrete anatomical structures and are invested by a partial capsule termed a hemicapsule. The surfacing epithelium may dip into the substance of the tonsils as crypts, foveolar pits or simple invaginations. The surfacing epithelium is often infiltrated with lymphocytes possibly to interact with antigens entering the body via the oropharynx through the nose or mouth. The tonsils do not contain a cortex and medulla but do contain lymphoid nodules and depending upon the state of stimulation these may contain germinal centers. There are three tonsilar groups. The paired palatine tonsils, located in the palatine fossa, are covered by stratified squamous epithelium and contain true crypts. The single pharyngeal tonsil is covered by pseudo-stratified columnar epithelium with cilia. Invagination of the surface epithelium into the depths of the organ as stratified squamous epithelium occurs but no true crypts are present. The lingual tonsils are located at the root of the tongue and are covered by the surface epithelium of the tongue, moist stratified squamous epithelium. Foveolar pits are present into which mucous glands may empty.

## CIRCULATORY SYSTEM

The circulatory system comprises both the cardiovascular and lymphatic systems. In common, these two systems comprise a series of closed tubular structures that transport fluid medium in which various types of cells are suspended. In the cardiovascular component of the circulatory system, blood, consisting of a fluid known as plasma and blood cells, circulates in a closed loop of endothelially lined vessels in which the heart is interposed to provide propulsive force. This arrangement provides a rapid movement of the blood throughout all parts of the body within closed circuits. The lymphatic system begins as blind endothelially lined vessels (lymphatic capillaries). The lymphatic vessels increase in size to eventually communicate with the cardiovascular system. Along the course of larger lymphatic vessels are interposed small organs of the immune system, the lymph nodes. Movement of fluid (lymph) and cells (chiefly lymphocytes) is dependent upon gravity and compression of the lymphatic vessels by surrounding tissues, i.e., skeletal muscle. Thus movement of lymph occurs slowly and unidirectionally from the periphery to the center of the body. Although the lymphatic system does not actually form a complete circuit, the structural similarities of its parts to those of the cardiovascular system and the direct anatomical communication between the two systems provide a basis for the integration of the two under a broader category, the circulatory system.

### Endothelium

The parenchyma of the circulatory system is a simple squamous epithelium known as endothelium. Endothelial structure varies largely with location and function. In the heart and large vessels, the endothelium is smooth to allow transport of blood or lymph with maximum efficiency. At the level of smaller vessels, particulary the capillaries, endothelial cells are modified in various ways to effect rapid exchange of gases, nutrients, fluid, waste metabolites or cells. Some endothelial cells function in other specialized roles, i.e., phagocytosis.

### Layers of the Circulatory System

The organs of the circulatory system (heart, arteries, veins, arterioles, venules and larger lymphatic vessels) are characterized by stromal elements which are arranged into three concentric layers or tunics about the functional parenchyma (endothelium).

1) Tunica intima - is the subluminal layer and consists of the endothelium, its basement membrane and a subendo-

thelial layer of connective tissue.

2) Tunica media - is the middle layer and the one most subject to structural modification in the various organs. Depending on the organ, the media may consist of smooth muscle, cardiac muscle, and various types of connective tissue including elastic connective tissue. The media is poorly represented or absent in some veins and totally lacking in capillaries. It is particularly specialized in the heart and large arteries.

3) Tunica adventitia or tunica serosa - is the outermost layer. It is generally composed of various types of connective tissue. Functionally, it may anchor the vessel into the surrounding tissue and in this configuration, it is referred to as the adventitia. Alternately, and depending on the location of the structure, it may be surfaced externally by a layer of simple squamous epithelium (mesothelium) in which case the term tunica serosa is applicable. The adventitial layer is particulary important in the larger vessels in that it carries the supporting stromal elements of these organs as small vessels (vasa vasorum) and nerves (vasa nervorum). In veins, the tunica adventitia or serosa is the most highly developed and functionally important layer. The adventitia of certain veins may contain fascicles of smooth muscle arranged parallel to the long axis of the vessel. This arrangement differs from the compact, circularly arranged smooth muscle in the media of muscular arteries and arterioles. The term tunica adventitia (or serosa) is generally not used in descriptions of capillaries.

## Heart

The heart is a modified, discrete region (an organ) of the circulatory system that is specialized for the propulsion of blood throughout the pulmonary and systemic circuits. Although it retains the same general organization of all the other organs of the circulatory system (arrangement into three layers or tunics), structural modifications of these allow it to carry out its specialized function. In the heart, the three layers receive an alternate and unique nomenclature. The tunica intima is termed the endocardium and in certain locations is modified as a redundant fold to form the cardiac valves. The endocardium of the atria is thicker than that of the ventricles. The tunica media is called the myocardium reflecting its chief component, striated cardiac muscle. The myocardium is highly vascularized by the coronary arteries and their branches. Special cardiac myocytes, the Purkinje cells may be found within the conducting pathways of the heart and are particularly prominent in the subendocardial layer. Purkinje cells are larger, stain lighter and contain more glycogen but fewer contractile myofilaments than the more abundant regular cardiac myocytes. The myocardium of the ventricles is thicker than that of the atria. The ventricular myocardium is more robust on the left side. The tunica serosa of the heart is referred to as the epicardium and consists of mesothelially covered connective tissue containing a variable amount of fat cells, blood vessels, ganglia (largely parasympathetic) and nerves.

The term cardiac skeleton refers to a connective tissue framework that serves as the site of origin and insertion of the atrial and ventricular musculature and as an attachment point for the atrioventricular valves (mitral and tricuspid).

## Arterial Vessels

Arterial vessels are distinguished histologically largely by the structure and components of the media. Depending upon the configuration of the media, these vessels may be designated as elastic arteries, muscular arteries or arterioles.

### Elastic Arteries

The tunica intima of elastic arteries is well-developed and easily visualized by light microscopy. The subendothelial connective tissue is delicate, contains collagen and elastic fibers and tends to blend imperceptibly with the middle and most prominent layer, the tunica media. The media of elastic arteries is composed of a concentric arrangement of multiple fenestrated elastic laminae (layers instead of fibers) alternating with layers of smooth muscle and connective tissue cells. In the proximal portions of large elastic arteries originating from the heart, cardiac muscle may be present in varying quantities. The tunica adventitia or, depending on the artery's proximity to a body cavity (pericardial, pleural or peritoneal), tunica serosa consists of areolar connective in which vasa vasorum and vasa nervorum may be found. These vessels and nerves supply the media which is much too thick to be supplied transmurally by luminal blood. Elastic arteries are conducting arteries which because of their elasticity function to buffer the fluctuations of blood pressure and flow which would otherwise occur during the cardiac cycle. Examples of elastic arteries include the aorta, pulmonary arteries, common iliacs and common carotids.

### Muscular Arteries

Muscular arteries include the named branches of elastic arteries, i.e. splenic, radial, etc. The tunica intima of muscular arteries is largely inconspicuous. The most prominent layer is the tunica media which is composed of a compact arrangement of many circularly or spirally disposed layers of smooth muscle cells. All muscular arteries are characterized by the presence of a well-developed internal elastic lamina which is considered to be the external part of the tunica intima but is probably synthesized by cells in the media. The adventitial layer of most muscular arteries is visually prominent and may equal the thickness of the media. It is often but not invariably demarcated from the underlying media by the presence an external elastic lamina. The tunica adventitia of muscular arteries contains vascular and nervous elements. The latter are particularly important in that they are vasomotor in nature. By stimulating contraction or relaxation of the smooth muscle in the media to effect a change in luminal size, the innervation of muscular arteries serves to regulate the flow of blood to dependent organs and tissues.

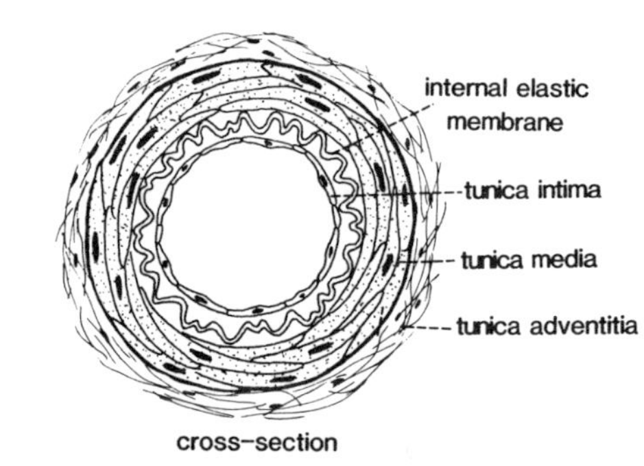


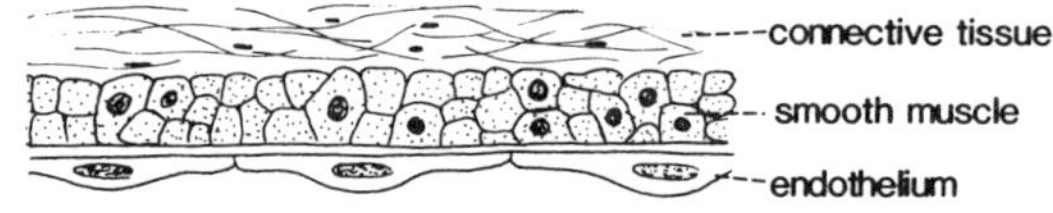


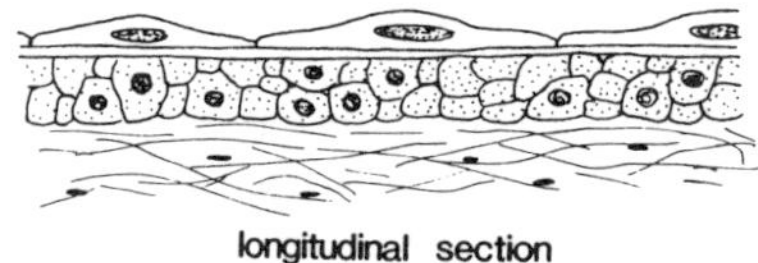


**Fig. 3.7.** Structure of a small artery.

## Arterioles

The smallest arterial organs are known as arterioles. They resemble small muscular arteries and are generally in the range of 20 to 100 microns in diameter. On a merely arbitrary basis, they can be distinguished from smaller muscular arteries by the number of layers of smooth muscle in the media. Using this criterion, small arteries that contain fewer than 5 layers of smooth muscle cells may be considered arterioles. In larger arterioles, an attenuated internal elastic lamina may be found while in the smaller ones it is entirely absent so that the tunica intima consists only of endothelium. The most conspicuous property of arterioles is that they appear relatively thick in comparison to their lumen. In the smallest arterioles (precapillary arterioles), a single layer of smooth muscle cells may comprise the media. The smooth muscle cells of the arteriolar media are the major regulators of systemic blood pressure. They may be innervated by vasomotor nerves found within the adventitia or in precapillary arterioles in which an adventitia and associated nervous elements may be lacking, circulating substances (i.e., catecholamines) diffusing from luminal blood may serve a vasomotor role.

## Venous Vessels

Venules, medium and large veins comprise the types of venous vessels. The variations that occur within each of these groups is greater than the differences encountered in the corresponding groups of arterial vessels. This classification does yield a working division of the types of vessels encountered on the venous side of the blood circulatory system.

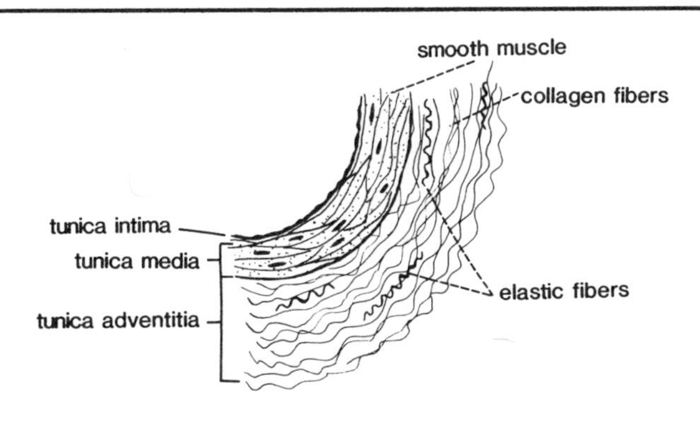


**Fig. 3.8.** Wall of a small vein.

### Venules

The smallest venules are thin walled structures which are only differentiated from capillaries by their larger size. Functionally, metabolic exchange may still occur in postcapillary venules. Gradually, stromal elements begin to accompany the endothelium, at first as only a thin, outer sheath of connective tissue. In venules with a diameter of 50 microns or greater, smooth muscle cells may be present as a media. They may be oriented in a circular arrangement as in arterioles but unlike them they do not form a compact layer. In so-called muscular venules, a media of 2 to 4 layers of widely spaced smooth muscle cells and a relatively thick adventitia containing fibroblasts, collagen and scattered elastic fibers is present.

## Medium Veins

Like muscular venules, medium-sized veins may contain a media of circularly arranged but widely spaced smooth muscle cells. The media of veins from the upper portions of the body tend to be less developed than that of comparably sized vessels from lower body regions. Medium sized veins often accompany muscular arteries (venae comitantes). The adventitia tends to be thicker than the media and may contain, in addition to fibroblasts, collagen fibers and elastic fibers, a few longitudinally arranged smooth muscle fibers. Medium-sized veins, particularly those of the lower extremities, may contain semilunar folds of intima (valves). Venous valves along with the more highly developed media present in certain veins below the heart function to resolve the problem of relatively high, gravity-generated venous pressure.

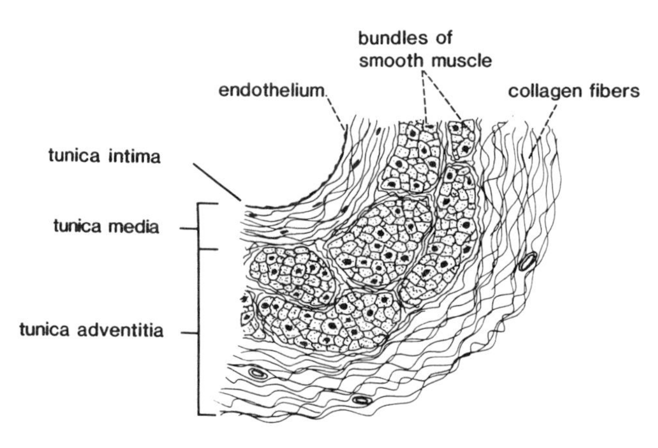


**Fig. 3.9.** Wall of a large vein.

## Large Veins

Veins of large caliber (superior and inferior venae cavae, portal vein and proximal tributaries) possess an unremarkable intima which is difficult to distinguish from the media. The media consists largely of connective tissue but circularly arranged, isolated smooth muscle cells may be present as well. The most characteristic feature of large veins is the presence of a well-developed and microscopically prominent tunica adventitia containing fascicles of longitudinally oriented smooth muscle cells. Cardiac muscle may extend for a distance within the serosa of the venae cavae and pulmonary veins in segments proximate to the heart.

## Capillaries

The arterial vessels function largely to transport the blood from the heart and to control the pressure and rate of delivery to the tissues and organs while the venous vessels return the blood to the heart. Interposed between the arterial and venous sides is a vast capillary network. It is at the capillary level that the major work of the circulatory system is performed. Capillaries are the smallest of arterial branches and generally are so small that red blood cells may pass through them one at a time. They consist of an endothelial tube and the abluminal basement membrane of the endothelial cells. Occasionally, small cells are located beneath the endothelial cell surrounded by its basement membrane. These cells are termed pericytes and are thought to function as reserve cells. The structure of capillaries is modified to conform with their varying functions. Three major types of capillaries exist.

### Continuous (Type I) Capillaries

This is the most common form. The endothelial cells of this type are joined along their outer edges by incomplete junctions (fascia occludens). Numerous pinocytotic vesicles are present in the endothelial cell cytoplasm indicating the mode of bidirectional interchange of fluid between capillary lumen and the extracapillary environment. This type of capillary is found in muscle and lungs. In the capillaries of the blood-brain barrier and blood-thymus barrier, the intercellular junctions are of the zonula occludens variety and pinocytotic vacuoles are sparse.

### Fenestrated (Type II) Capillaries

This form is also considered a continuous type because the basement membrane is continuous. They differ from those described above in that the endothelial cells contain numerous pits or pores with a diameter of approximately 70 nm. The pores represent foci of attenuated cytoplasm. In most fenestrated capillaries, a thin diaphragm (thinner than the endothelial plasma membrane) spans the fenestra. In others, the diaphragm is absent so that the fenestrations truly represent transcellular holes. Fenestrated capillaries with diaphragms occur in the intestinal villi, endocrine organs, choroid plexi and ciliary body. Those without diaphragms are found in the renal glomeruli. The proposed function of the fenestrations and diaphragms is to provide a rapid but somewhat selective transport of fluid and solutes across the endothelium.

## Discontinuous Capillaries

These are also termed sinusoidal capillaries or sometimes simply sinusoids. They are irregular in shape and possess large intercellular gaps between which fluid (plasma) and cells may pass readily. The gaps are often occupied by macrophages. In the liver, the endothelial cells of the sinusoids may function as sessile macrophages and are termed Kupffer cells. Besides the liver, discontinuous capillaries are the predominate type present in spleen and bone marrow. The basement membrane is incomplete (discontinuous) or in some instances absent.

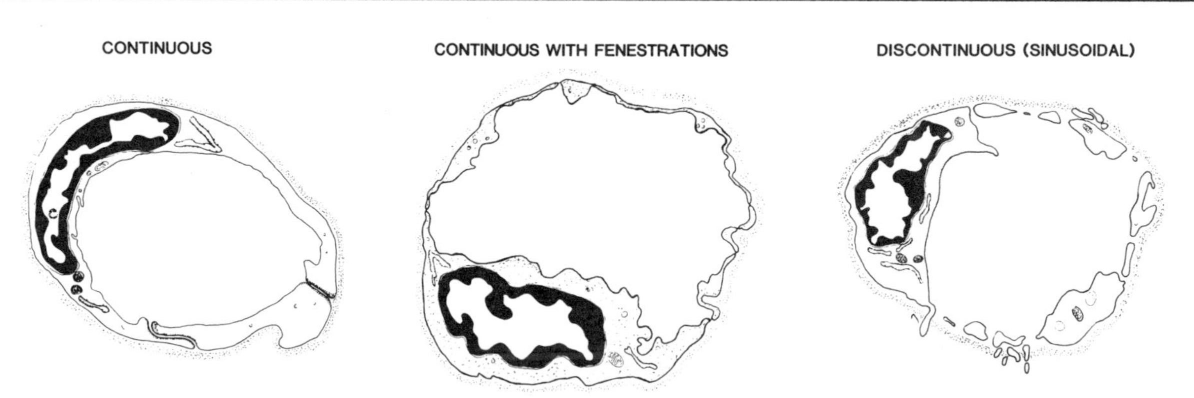


Fig. 3.10. Different types of capillaries.

## Lymphatic Vessels

The lymphatic limb of the circulatory system begins as blind-ended or looped capillaries located throughout many tissues and organs. Lymphatic capillaries tend to be larger in diameter than blood capillaries and to vary in size along their course. For the most part the endothelium is continuous. Definite gaps may occur between adjacent endothelial cells and pinocytotic vacuoles may be found within the cytoplasm. With increasing diameter, the lymphatic vessels eventually acquire the three characteristic tunics found in other components of the circulatory system. The intima of larger conducting lymphatic vessels consists of the endothelium and a thin, subjacent layer of elastic and collagenous fibers. Valves may be present. The media may contain a few layers of spirally arranged smooth muscle fibers. The adventitia is the thickest layer and consists of a collagen and elastic fiber network in which a small number of smooth muscle cells may be found. The main lymphatic trunks (thoracic and right lymphatic ducts) contain a prominent media in which both longitudinal and circular bundles of smooth muscle may be found. The intima may contain a thin, but inconstant elastic membrane. The adventitia is unremarkable.

# ENDOCRINE SYSTEM

The endocrine system consists of a group of glands which are structurally and functionally related. Each produces one or more secretory products (hormones) that are released into the vascular system which disseminates the hormones to the various target tissues and organs on which they act. This functional aspect is reflected by the relative rich vascular supply associated with most of the endocrine glands. In most, but not all the endocrine organs, transitory ducts are present during development which are subsequently lost. Exceptions include the adrenals and the endocrine portions of the male and female sex glands. Individual endocrine glands are developmentally derived from one of any of the three primary germ layers: endoderm, ectoderm or mesoderm. Those glands developing from ectoderm or endoderm produce protein or protein-related hormones (amino acid derivatives, polypeptides, simple or complex proteins). Mesodermally derived endocrine organs produce steroid hormones. The endocrine components of the gonads will be discussed in the appropriate sections of the male and female reproductive systems and the endocrine portion of the pancreas will be presented in conjunction with its exocrine function in the section on the digestive system.

## Pituitary Gland

Also called the hypophysis cerebri, this organ consists of two main components, the adenohypophysis and the neurohypophysis. The neurohypophysis functions in conjunction with the hypothalamus. The adenohypophysis is often subdivided into three parts: pars distalis, pars tuberalis and pars intermedia. The neurohypophysis consists of the pars nervosa and infundibulum. The infundibulum may be further subdivided into the infundibular stem and the median eminence of the tuber cinereum. Additionally, the pituitary may be divided into an anterior and posterior lobe. The former consists of the pars distalis and pars tuberalis while the latter is composed of pars intermedia and pars nervosa. Secretions of the anterior lobe are protein in nature.

### Adenohypophysis

The glandular cells of the adenohypophysis may be classified as chromophils or chomophobes based on their staining patterns with routine techniques like hematoxylin and eosin. By electron microscopy, cytoplasmic granules which vary in size from cell to cell are present in all chromophils and to a lesser degree in many chromophobes. Chromophils contain specific granules that stain either basophilic (basophils) or eosinophilic (acidophils). The PAS reaction also stains the specific granules of basophils because these granules are composed in part of carbohydrate. The nature of chromophobes is still somewhat controversial. They were once considered reserve cells that are devoid of specific granules but capable of differentiating into either acidophils or basophils. More recent evidence indicates that at least some chromophobes simply represent either acidophils or basophils that have recently undergone degranulation and thus the differentiating feature (specific granules) is not present for absolute identification. By electron microscopy and immunohistochemical techniques, very few cells prove to be totally unidentifiable as either a type of acidophil or a type of basophil.

### Acidophils

These cells are also known as alpha cells. Their specific granules stain with eosin but not with PAS. Two specific types occur which are differentiated by the specific hormone secreted. They are termed somatotrophs and mammotrophs.

1) Somatotrophs - secrete somatotropin (STH, growth hormone or GH). GH stimulates many tissues including (via somatomedin) the cartilaginous tissue of the epiphyseal plates of long bones. Human pituitary gigantism and acromegaly are caused by acidophil tumors of the pars distalis. A deficiency of somatotrophs results in pituitary dwarfism. Somatotrophs may be demonstrated by specific immunohistochemical staining methods.

2) Mammotrophs - secrete prolactin which initiates and maintains milk production in the post-partal female. Immunohistochemical methods are available.

### Basophils

Also termed beta-cells, these cells stain poorly but basophilic with hematoxylin. Because of the carbohydrate moiety of the specific granules, PAS staining is more intense and thus more reliable for their identification. There are three types of basophils. Immunohistochemical methods are available for localizing many of the hormones produced by basophils.

1) Corticotrophs - secrete ACTH and lipotrophic hormone (beta-LPH). Actually, they produce a 31,000 molecular weight prohormone (pro-opiomelanocortin) that undergoes post-translational cleavage to yield ACTH and LPH. LPH may be further metabolized to produce beta-endorphin, an opiate-like polypeptide, and melanocyte stimulating hormone (MSH).

2) Thyrotrophs - also termed beta-basophils, they secrete TSH which is stimulatory for the follicular cells of the thyroid. These cells contain the smallest granules

of any of the chromophils. Thyrotrophs are said to stain specifically with aldehyde fuchsin.

3) Gonadotrophs - alternately termed delta-basophils, they secrete the gonadotrophins, FSH and LH. FSH stimulates development of ovarian follicles in the female and in the male initiates spermatogenesis at puberty. LH stimulates estrogen secretion by developing ovarian follicles and in the male, it promotes testosterone secretion by the interstitial cells (Leydig) of the testis. For this reason LH in the male is often termed interstitial cell stimulating hormone (ICSH). Immunohistochemical staining reveals that some gonadotrophs produce LH, others produce FSH and some apparently produce both hormones.

## Neurohypophyseal Complex

The neurohypophyseal complex consists of portions of the hypothalamus, the median eminence of the tuber cinereum, the infundibular stem and the infundibular process (pars nervosa). All the releasing factors and hormones associated with the neurohypophyseal complex are formed by neurons located in the hypothalamus and secreted by their axon terminals in the posterior lobe of the pituitary. Two main neuronal secretory systems exit.

1) Parvicellular system - axons from hypothalamic neurons extend to the median eminence where secretion of the various releasing and inhibiting factors which control the rate of release of the adenohypophyseal hormones occurs.

2) Magnocellular neurosecretory system - the unmyelinated axons of neurons within the supraoptic and paraventricular nuclei form the hypothalamohypophyseal tract. This system produces and secretes two hormones: oxytocin and vasopressin. Oxytocin stimulates contraction of the myometrium of the pregnant uterus during parturition and promotes the ejection of milk in the lactating breast. Vasopressin (ADH) increases the permeability of the kidney collecting ducts to water so that most of the water in the filtrate is reabsorbed.

## Pituicytes

These cells are located in the posterior lobe and form a three-dimensional network with neighboring cells. Long processes of pituicytes join end to end with those of others and communicate via gap junctions. The pituicytes are analogous to astrocytes of the CNS proper and their proposed function is to support and provide metabolic maintenance of the secretory axon terminals.

**Thyroid Gland**

The thyroid is surrounded by a thin connective tissue capsule from which septae extend into the gland to incompletely divide it into lobules. The major parenchymal cells are organized into spherical structures termed follicles. Follicles are cyst-like structures consisting of a single layer of secretory epithelial cells surrounding a central mass of gelatinous material, the colloid. In humans, the follicles are barely perceptible to the naked eye and measure 0.02 to 0.9 mm in diameter. Rich blood and lymphatic capillary plexuses are present in the connective tissue which separates individual follicles. The follicular cells rest on a basement membrane which is visualized only at the electron microscopic level. Follicular cells vary in height from columnar to squamous depending on their state of functional activity. Two types of cells may be found within the follicles.

1) Follicular cells - comprise the vast majority of the cells within the follicles. They are arranged in a single layer resting on a basement membrane with their apices directed inward toward the follicular cavity. Cells in actively secreting follicles are columnar while inactive follicles are lined by a squamous layer. Nuclei are generally spherical with one or more prominent nucleoli. At the light microscopic level, a supranuclear Golgi complex, lipid droplets and PAS-positive material may be observed in the usually basophilic cytoplasm. Ultrastructurally, the active cells (columnar to cuboidal) contain typical junctional complexes at the apical portion of the lateral plasma membranes. Short microvilli may be observed on the apical borders and numerous profiles of RER are located in the basal region. The cytoplasm contains abundant lysosomes and multivesicular bodies. Membrane-bound bodies in the apical region are termed colloidal resorption droplets. The follicular cells secrete: thyroglobulin into the colloid and thyroid hormones ($T_3$ and $T_4$) into the surrounding blood and lymphatic capillaries.

2) Parafollicular cells - also termed C cells, they occur as single cells and small cell groups located within the follicular epithelium (on the colloid side of the basement membrane) or may be scattered within the connective tissue between follicles. When located within the basement membrane they are usually located very near it and do not extend to the follicular lumen. They have a different embryologic origin than the follicular cells and secrete thyrocalcitonin. Ultra-

structurally, they contain numerous membrane-bound secretory granules measuring 0.1 to 0.5 microns in diameter which have been shown by immunocytochemical methods to be thyrocalcitonin.

Colloid

The thyroid gland is unique among the endocrine glands in that it stores large quantities of hormones in an inactive form within extracellular compartments (colloid) in contrast to other endocrine glands which store only small amounts of hormone intracellularly. Colloid stains with both basic and acidic dyes and is PAS-positive. It consists of proteolytic enzymes, mucoproteins and the glycoprotein, thyroglobulin. Active resorption of the colloid by follicular cells results in a vacuolated, scalloped appearance at the interface of the follicular cells with the colloidal material. Colloid resorbed by follicular cells is used to produce iodinated polypeptide hormones which are secreted into the vascular system and circulate as free or protein-bound (bound to thyroid-binding globulin or thyroid-binding prealbumen) molecules of triiodothyronine ($T_3$) or thyroxine ($T_4$) in a $T_4/T_3$ ratio of 20:1.

## Parathyroid Glands

Usually represented by two pairs of small (50 mg each) glands embedded within the connective tissue capsule on the posterior surface of the thyroid. Each glandular mass is surrounded by a thin connective tissue capsule from which extend septae that partially divide it into poorly defined lobules. The parenchymal cells are densely packed and are arranged into anastomosing cords separated by vascular spaces and connective tissue. A few fat cells may be present within the connective tissue stroma early in life. The number of adipocytes increases dramatically at puberty and continues to increase throughout life so that in elderly adults 60-70% of the glandular mass may be fat. The parathyroids produce the polypeptide hormone, parathormone (PTH). There are two types of parenchymal cells present within the parathyroid glands.

1) Principal or chief cells - are small polygonal cells measuring approximately 7-10 microns in diameter. They contain a centrally placed, vesicular nucleus and a pale-staining, slightly acidophilic cytoplasm. Ultrastructurally, lipofuscin granules, glycogen granules, lipid droplets and small, dense membrane-limited granules may be seen.

2) Oxyphil cells - constitute a minor portion of the parenchymal cells. They appear first at age 7-10 and become relatively more abundant with increasing age. They are distinctly larger than chief cells and have an

intensely staining eosinophilic cytoplasm. The nuclei tend to be smaller than those of chief cells and contain more heterochromatin. They occur as single cells or as small groups surrounded by the predominant chief cells. Ultrastructurally, numerous mitochondria are present which correlates with the cytoplasmic acidophilia apparent by light microscopy. The cytoplasm contains a limited amount of ER, a small Golgi apparatus and normally no secretory granules. Their function is not known.

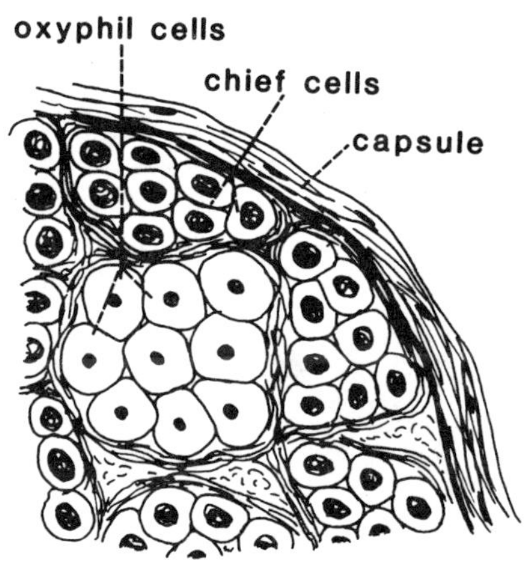


**Fig. 3.11.** Parathyroid.

### Adrenal Glands

The adrenal glands are structurally and functionally composite organs. They are divided into a cortex and medulla which differ in their structure, function and developmental origin. Both are considered to be endocrine in function but the hormones produced are quite different. The cortex produces a variety of steroid hormones and is of mesodermal origin. The medulla is derived from neural crest and secretes catecholamines.

#### Cortex

The cortex consists of three zones that form concentric layers about the central medulla.

1) The outer <u>zona glomerulosa</u> comprises about 15% of the cortical volume. The cells are arranged into irregular, ovoid clusters. The secretory cells have darkly-staining spherical nuclei and little cytoplasm. By EM,

the cytoplasm shows SER, numerous mitochondria and small lipid droplets. The cells produce mineralocorticoids, particularly aldosterone, and are largely independent of ACTH stimulation.

2) The middle zona fasciculata is the thickest layer and contributes about 75% of the cortical volume. The cells are polyhedral in shape and arranged in long, narrow cords one to two cells thick. Adjacent cords are separated by sinusoidal blood vessels. The cells often have a foamy appearance which by EM proves to be due to numerous cytoplasmic lipid droplets. Profiles of SER and mitochondria containing tubular cristae are particularly abundant. A well-developed Golgi apparatus is also observable. This zone is ACTH-dependent and is stimulated to produce and secrete glucocorticoids, especially cortisone, and normally small quantities of sex hormones.

3) The innermost zona reticularis comprises approximately 10% of the cortical volume. The cells are similar in appearance to those of the zone above but the cords are much shorter and tend to anastomose with each other. They do differ in that they contain few lipid droplets but abundant lipofuscin pigment. This layer, like the one above, is dependent upon ACTH and secretes glucocorticoids and lesser amounts of sex hormones.

## Medulla

When the adrenal gland is fixed in solutions containing chromium salts (dichromate anions), the cells of the adrenal medulla which contain catecholamines stain brown, the so-called chromaffin reaction. In aldehyde-fixed material, the granules also result in autoflourescence of some of the cells. The cells of the medulla are innervated by preganglionic sympathetic fibers which stimulate the release of the granules that contain either norepinephrine or epinephrine. The cells are divided into two types on the basis of the structure of the membrane-bound granules that they produce. Those cells that store norepinephrine possess cytoplasmic granules with an electron-dense core while epinephrine storing cells have granules that are less electron dense.

# INTEGUMENTARY SYSTEM

## General Comments

The integument consists of the skin that covers the surface of the body along with specialized skin derivatives. These include:

1) Hair
2) Nails
3) Glands
   a) Sebaceous glands
   b) Sweat glands
      i) Eccrine
      ii) Apocrine
   c) Mammary glands

The skin is composed of two layers, the epidermis and below it the dermis. The dermis eventually blends into the underlying hypodermis (subcutis) which corresponds to the superficial fascia of gross anatomy. The hypodermis is not considered part of the skin although adnexal structures may be found there. The epidermis is of ectodermal origin and consists of a keratinized stratified squamous epithelium while the dermis is a vascularized dense irregular fibrous connective tissue of mesodermal origin.

External examination of the skin reveals a free surface exhibiting numerous free ridges observable with the naked eye. These surface markings are most apparent on the palms and soles as loops, whorls and arches (dermatoglyphics). Their pattern is determined largely by hereditary factors. Where an epidermal ridge is present externally, a narrow projection, the rete ridge, is present on the dermal aspect. On either side of the rete ridge, dermal papillae project irregularly into the epidermis. Dermal papillae are numerous, tall, often branched and most notable where the epidermis is thick.

### Thick and Thin Skin

A thick epidermis is present normally on palms and soles; thin skin is found elsewhere. The dermis of extensor surfaces is usually thicker than that of flexor surfaces.

## Epidermis

There are four distinct cell types present in the epidermis. They are: keratinocytes, Merkel cells, melanocytes and Langerhans cells. The keratinocytes are of ectodermal origin while the melanocytes and Merkel cells are derived from neural crest ectoderm. Langerhans cells are probably of bone marrow origin and are related to the monocyte/macrophage system. The most numerous cell of the epidermis is the keratinocyte, so named because in its fully differentiated state it produces the protein keratin. The structural organization of the epidermis into layers (stratified epithelium) reflects stages in the life cycle of the keratinocyte. This cycle involves cellular proliferation and growth, outward displacement and differentiation, death and finally desquamation into the external environment.

The layers of the epidermis are maximally represented in the thick skin. The layers in order from the basement membrane upward and a brief description of each follows:

## Stratum basale

More commonly known as the basal layer, other synonymous appellations include: stratum germinativum and stratum cylindricum. It consists of a single layer of cuboidal or low columnar cells with thin cytoplasmic processes on the basal surface which fit into corresponding pockets within the basal lamina that serve as anchoring points. Hemidesmosomes are also present on the basal surface and desmosomes are seen on lateral and superior surfaces. Fine (intermediate) filaments known as tonofilaments are distributed throughout the cytoplasm which when present as aggregates (tonofibrils) can be seen by light microscopy. Mitotic figures, indicating the proliferative role of this layer, can often be found.

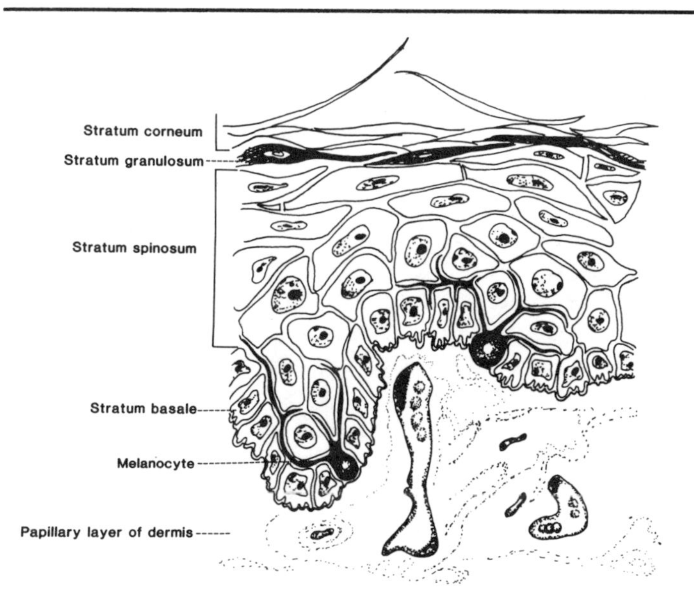


**Fig. 3.12.** Epidermal layers.

## Stratum spinosum

This layer is also known as the prickle cell layer and is

several cell layers thick. The cells (spinocytes) are irregular, polygonally-shaped cells which by light microscopy appear slightly separated from each other and covered by short cytoplasmic extensions which meet with similar projections of adjacent cells. These structures are referred to as intercellular bridges and are due to two things. The first is artifactual shrinkage of the cells which increases the intercellular space and the second is the presence of rigid points of attachment (desmosomes) between adjacent cells which prevent separation of the cell membranes at those points only. The keratinocytes of the stratum spinosum also contain tonofilaments and stain basophilic reflecting their RNA content associated with protein synthesis for growth and division of the cells. NOTE: the stratum basale in combination with the stratum germinativum is sometimes called the stratum Malpighii. This layer contains the before mentioned cells as well as other epidermal cells, i.e., Merkel cells, melanocytes and Langerhans cells.

## Stratum granulosum

The stratum granulosum is more commonly known as the granular layer. It consists of 2 to 5 layers of flattened cell with their long axis oriented parallel to the skin surface. Their name derives from the presence of cytoplasmic granules of keratohyalin which stain intensely with hematoxylin. By electron microscopy they are irregular masses of electron-dense material present in association with bundles of filaments. The granules are probably involved in the formation of "soft keratin". NOTE: Soft keratin is associated with the skin proper whereas hard keratin is found in the nails and hair. They differ in that the latter contains more sulfur.

The stratum granulosum is the site where degenerative changes of the nucleus may be first discerned or in other words the cells begin to die in this layer. The keratinocytes of the granular layer, as well of those of upper portions of the stratum spinosum, may also contain small "membrane-coating granules". Also known as keratinosomes or Odland bodies, they are formed in association with the Golgi apparatus from which they move to the periphery of the cell in order to discharge their contents into the intercellular space. The extruded material is thought to function as a barrier to penetration by foreign materials and is particularly impervious to water. This is particularly important since the superficial and underlying layers are fairly permeable to water.

## Stratum lucidum

This layer is difficult to distinguish except in the epidermis of thick skin. Typically it is composed of a clear, translucent layer, 3 to 5 cells in thickness in the thick skin with a lesser thickness in thin skin. The cells are not distinguishable as separate entities because they are extremely flattened, mostly anuclear and closely packed. The cytoplasm contains keratohyalin, presumably a product of granules in subjacent layers, distributed among the tonofibrils which lie in a parallel arrangement to the skin surface.

## Stratum corneum

This is the fully differentiated, functional layer of the skin. It is composed of clear, dead cells which are flattened and fused. The nuclei are absent and the cytoplasm is filled with keratin of tonofilament origin. In hematoxylin and eosin strained sections, the stratum corneum is quite obvious and stains pink distinguishing it from the various degrees of basophilia noted in subjacent layers. The most superficial cells are constantly desquamating and in aggregate the outermost layers are called the stratum disjunctum.

## The Melanocyte and Pigmentation

Developmentally, melanocytes are derived from the neural crest. They are found in the stratum basale and to a lesser extent, the stratum spinosum. They are also associated with hair follicles. The melanocyte has a dendritic appearance and lacks desmosomes and tonofilaments. The dendritic processes are observed to extend between adjacent keratinocytes. As their name implies, melanocytes produce the pigment melanin. Formation of melanin occurs within membrane-bound granules termed melanosomes. Melanosomes contain tyrosinase, an enzyme synthesized in ribosomes and subsequently transferred by the endoplasmic reticulum to the Golgi where it is packaged into vesicles which fuse with the premelanosomes. Thus tyrosinase is present in melanosomes but not in premelanosomes. The maturation of the melanosome is complex and several morphologic stages are noted at the ultrastructural level. Once mature, they are transferred to the keratinocytes of the stratum germinativum and stratum spinosum by a somewhat controversial mechanism.

Melanocytes are difficult to identify with certainty in conventionally stained preparations. The dopa reaction can be used to ascertain their presence and location in tissue and culture if tyrosinase-containing melanosomes are present. Melanocytes are influenced by an anterior pituitary hormone, melanocyte stimulating hormone (MSH), which stimulates both the migration of mature melanosomes into the dendritic processes and the transfer of the granules to keratinocytes.

## Langerhans Cell

The Langerhans cell is a stellate-shaped (dendritic) cell located within the stratum spinosum. By light microscopy they appear as clear cells; their dendritic nature is only apparent after metal impregnation, especially with gold chloride methods.

In electron micrographs, they are seen to possess an indented nucleus with a relatively clear cytoplasm. Specifically absent are tonofilaments, desmosomes and melanosomes. Cytoplasmic inclusions which have the appearance of a tennis racket (Birbeck granules) are present which aids in their identification at the ultrastructural level.

Its origin is probably from bone marrow and is of immunological importance. It is thought to represent an antigen processing cell (APC) and is likely related to the cells of the monocyte/macrophage system.

### Merkel Cell

This cell has a fairly wide epithelial distribution but most commonly is found in or near the basal layer often in association with intraepithelial nerve endings, the so-called Merkel cell-neurite complex. The Merkel cell is not reliably recognized by routine light microscopy but can be visualized by use of silver impregnation techniques. Sections of skin prepared in this manner reveal the presence of a meniscoid neural terminal covering the basal portion of each Merkel cell. These are sometime referred to as Merkel's disks. A sensory nerve fiber terminates at each disk. The location of the Merkel cell is irregular and it is occasionally seen with others in small groups. It is thought to represent a mechanoreceptor.

## Dermis

The dermis ranges from 0.5 to 5.0 mm in thickness and merges imperceptibly into the underlying hypodermis. Upward projections of the dermis are seen as the so-called dermal papillae which interdigitate with the downward projecting rete ridges of the epidermis. The dermis is composed of two layers segregated by position and density of collagen fibers. The papillary layer lies between the epidermal basement membrane above and the underlying reticular dermis. It surrounds all the appendageal structures as they extend downward into the reticular dermis and hypodermis. As its name implies, it constitutes the core of the dermal papillae. Some papillae contains prominent loops of capillaries (vascular papillae) while other harbor special nerve endings (nervous papillae). Structurally, the papillary dermis consists of thin collagenous, reticular and elastic fibers embedded within ground substance. The second layer is called the reticular layer and lies immediately below the papillary layer. It comprises the main fibrous bed of the dermis and consists of dense irregular connective tissue in which a few reticular and numerous elastic fibers may be found. Appendages of the skin, when present, are located within the reticular dermis or at the junction of the reticular dermis and the hypodermis. Other cells and structures which may be present include: fibroblasts, migratory connective tissue cells, smooth muscle cells (arrector pili) and in certain anatomic regions, skeletal muscle (i.e., platysma).

## Nails

The nails are horny plates that form a protective covering on the dorsal surface of the terminal phalanges of the fingers and toes. Each nail consists of three parts:

1) Body - the attached, visible portion.
2) Free edge - the outward unattached extension of the body.
3) Nail root - the proximal portion which is covered by skin.

The epidermis directly beneath the nail is termed the nail bed while the skin in contact with the proximal and lateral border of the nail constitutes the nail fold. The nail bed and nail fold (wall) meet in the region of a narrow U-shaped furrow, the nail groove. While the larger, distal portion of the nail body is translucent and pink because of the underlying blood vessels, its most proximal part is represented by a whitish crescent-shaped area, the lunule. The epidermis of the nail bed is continuous distally with the undersurface of the free edge at the hyponychium. The stratum corneum of the skin extends over the proximal nail fold onto the free surface of the nail body at the eponychium or cuticle. The nail body consists of tightly packed keratinized cells produced by the underlying matrix, a mitotically-active derivative of the epidermis.

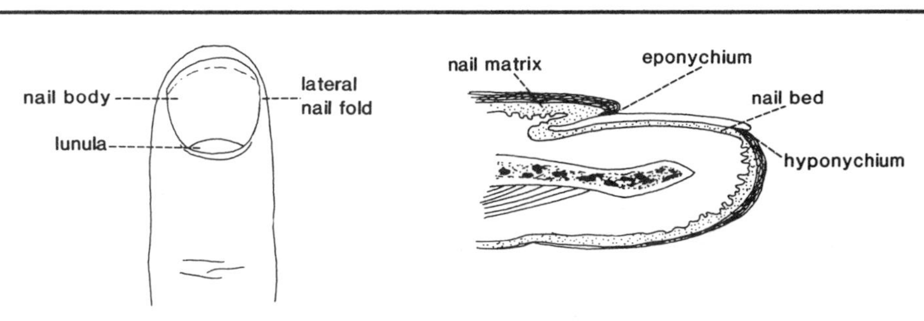


**Fig. 3.13.** Structure of the nail.

## Hair

Hairs are elastic, keratinized filamentous projections that develop from the epidermis. They are found everywhere except the palms, soles, dorsal distal phalanges, anal and urogenital openings. A hair is composed of a free shaft and a root embedded in the skin. Enclosing the hair root is a tubular hair follicle which is composed of epidermal (epithelial) and dermal (connective tissue) portions. The lower end of the follicle expands into a bulb which is indented at its basal end by a connective tissue papillae. Associated with most hair follicles are one or more sebaceous glands and a smooth muscle bundle, the arrector pili. The hair shaft and its associated sebaceous gland(s) constitute the pilosebaceous unit. There is no correlation between diameter of the hair shaft and the size or number of the sebaceous glands in the pilosebaceous unit. In fact, some of the larger sebaceous glands are associated with very fine hairs (vellus hairs).

## Glands of the Skin

The glands of the skin are derivatives of the epidermis as are the other cutaneous appendages. These glands include the sebaceous type, two kinds of sweat glands (eccrine and apocrine) and the mammary glands. Sebaceous glands most often develop from the outer root sheath of hair germs. Sweat glands originate as solid cords of epithelial cells that grow downward into the dermis. The distal portion becomes thickened and coiled to become the secretory portion. Initially the secretory portion and its duct are solid but later canalization produces a lumen. The mammary glands develop as epidermal thickenings in the site of the definitive nipple. Proliferation, downward growth and lateral extension of the epithelium results in a roughly hemispheric mass with a convex surface interfaced with the surrounding dermis. Subsequently some 20 primitive ducts, that are first solid and later canalized, form and begin to branch. Each of these contributes a separate lobe which connects to the surface at the nipple via a duct. At puberty further ductal development and the accumulation of fat occurs. The glandular component (alveoli) develop during pregnancy from small interlobular ducts which with corresponding secretory alveoli constitute numerous lobules within each lobe.

### Sebaceous Glands

The sebaceous glands are usually associated with hair follicles and are not present on the palms and soles. Notable exceptions where the glands empty directly onto the surface include the lips (Fordyce spots), oral and buccal mucosa, areolae and nipples (Montgomery's tubercles), labia minora, glans penis and prepuce (Tyson's glands). The meibomian glands of the eyelids are also of the sebaceous type and are not connected with hair follicles. They are simple, branched alveolar glands which secrete by the holocrine method. They may be unilobular or multilobular. At the periphery of each lobule, roughly cuboid-shaped cells differentiate into large, vacuolated lipid-laden cells. These disintegrate as they reach the duct which is composed of stratified squamous epithelium.

# CUTANEOUS APPENDAGES

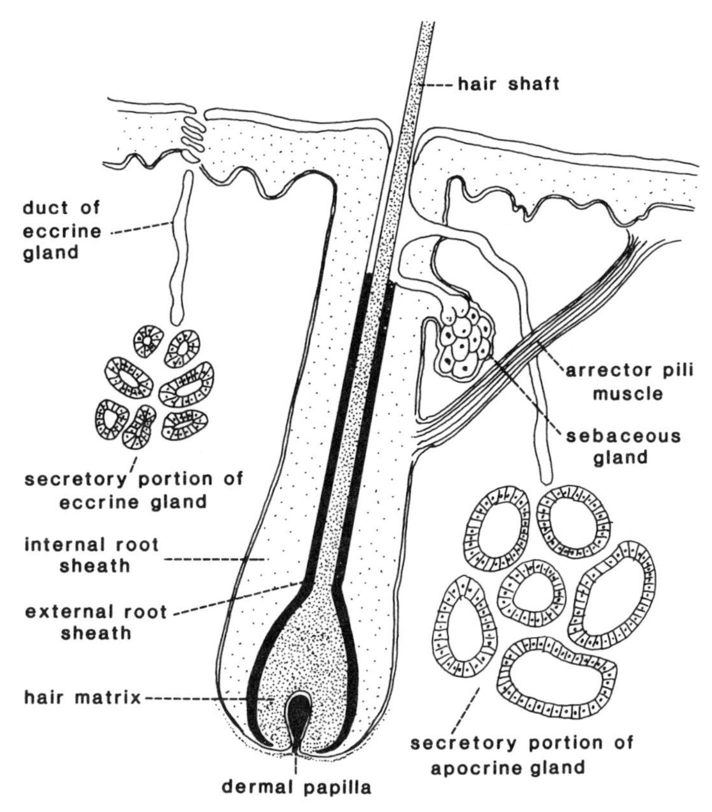


**Fig. 3.14.** Adnexal skin strucures.

## Sweat Glands

There are two types of sweat glands that differ in the composition of their secretory product. They can easily be differentiated morphologically by the difference in the size of the secretory lumen. The two types are eccrine and apocrine.

### Eccrine Glands

These produce a watery substance, which when modified by the ducts is expressed to the surface as sweat. They are especially numerous on the palms and soles, axillae and forehead. They are present nearly throughout the integument except the nail beds, earlobes and mucocutaneous junctions. The gland consists of a secretory portion which is located deep within the dermis or upper hypodermis and a duct. The duct may be defined as two portions, an intradermal part and an intraepithelial part. Structurally, the eccrine gland is a simple unbranched highly coiled tubular gland whose duct opens onto the surface of the skin at a sweat pore.

## Apocrine Glands

The secretions of apocrine glands are considered odiferous, a property which is dependent on bacterial action. They are most numerous in the axillae and groin but may be present on the scalp, forehead, areolae, circumanal and periumbilical regions as well. Other glands which are considered to be of apocrine derivation are the mammary glands, ceruminous glands of the auditory canal and Moll's glands of the eyelids. The secretory unit is located within the hypodermis and is differentiated from the eccrine type by relatively large lumina. Secretion is by the apocrine mode as their name indicates. Secretory material contains stainable iron granules and lysozyme can be demonstrated histochemically. The ducts, like those of most sebaceous glands, may open into the infundibulum of hair follicles above the sebaceous duct orifice or directly onto the skin surface.

## Mammary Glands

The mammary gland, a compound tubulo-alveolar exocrine gland, is considered to be a modified sweat gland of the apocrine type which is largely under hormonal control. As such, it develops within the superficial fasciae from the overlying epithelium. Each gland consists of approximately 20 lobes connected to the nipple by a lactiferous duct which dilates at the apex of the nipple into a lactiferous sinus. The lobes are separated by interlobar septae composed of dense irregularly oriented bundles of collagen mixed with elastic fibers which continues into the lobes between lobules as interlobular connective tissue. The histologic appearance of the mammary gland depends upon its state of maturity and actively so that a different morphologic picture is present in the juvenile, mature inactive and mature lactating breast.

1) Juvenile breast - ducts are the principal epithelial component. Intralobular ducts are grouped into small "lobules" separated from adjacent dense irregular connective tissue (interlobar and interlobular) by a notable layer of subepithelial areolar connective tissue. The lining of the ducts is stratified (2-4 layers) and true secretory alveoli are absent although gland-like buds composed of more than one cell layer may be seen.

2) Mature inactive breast - under the influence of hormones at puberty the breasts enlarge, partially by continued branching of the ductal system but mostly by the appearance of masses of adipose tissue within the interlobular connective tissue. Secretory alveoli, as in the juvenile breast, are absent.

3) Lactating breast - during the first half of pregnancy, the intralobular ducts undergo rapid proliferation and buds form which enlarge into alveoli. During the second half of pregnancy, well-developed lobules containing recognizable alveoli and intralobular ducts are present. Interlobular connective tissue decreases in amount. The alveoli are lined by simple columnar epithelial cells. Myoepithelial cells are associated with the secretory and ductal epithelium. Secretion of a serous fluid known as colostrum occurs in the third trimester but milk production does not occur until 2 to 3 days post-partum. The alveoli of the post-partal lactating breast are abundant and many are filled with secretory material with a vacuolated appearance although others may be empty.

# RESPIRATORY SYSTEM

There are two main divisions of the respiratory system. The air conduction division includes the nasal cavity, nasopharynx, larynx, trachea, bronchi and bronchioles. The respiratory division is modified for an efficient bidirectional exchange of gases between the blood and inspired air. This portion includes the respiratory bronchioles, alveolar ducts, alveolar sacs and alveoli.

## Upper Respiratory Tract

The nasal cavity, paranasal sinuses, nasopharynx and larynx contain an epithelial lining of pseudostratified columnar cells with cilia and associated goblet cells. Mixed seromucous glands are present in the underlying connective tissue. Since this type of epithelium is common in both the upper and lower respiratory tracts, it is often referred to simply as respiratory epithelium. This epithelium is modified in the olfactory portion of the nasal cavity and is termed olfactory mucosa. It will be addressed in a subsequent section on special senses. The epithelial membrane of the rest of the nasal cavity is called respiratory mucosa and functions to conduct, warm, moisten and partially cleanse the inspired air.

The respiratory epithelium of the nasopharynx is often interrupted by the oropharyngeal epithelium of stratified squamous cells (moist stratified squamous epithelium). The pharyngeal tonsil (adenoids) is present in the posterior wall.

The larynx is covered superiorly by the epiglottis containing a plate of elastic cartilage. The larynx connects the pharynx with the trachea. It contains both hyaline (thyroid, cricoid and arytenoids) and elastic (corniculates, cuneiforms and tips of the arytenoids) cartilages. Also present are the vocal cords which function in phonation.

## Lower Respiratory Tract

The lower respiratory tract consists of the trachea, bronchi and lungs. Conduction of air without gaseous exchange begins with the trachea and follows through a series of branching tubes which decrease in diameter with each successive order. Sixteen generations of dichotomous branching occur between the trachea and the final conducting tubes, the terminal bronchioles. Although imprecise, it is common to refer to the successive conducting branches of the trachea in order of their generation simply as bronchi, bronchioles and terminal bronchioles.

### Trachea and Primary Bronchi

The trachea is a relatively large (about 2 cm diameter)

flexible tube. It is supported by some 16 to 20 U-shaped cartilages of the hyaline type. The posterior free edges of the

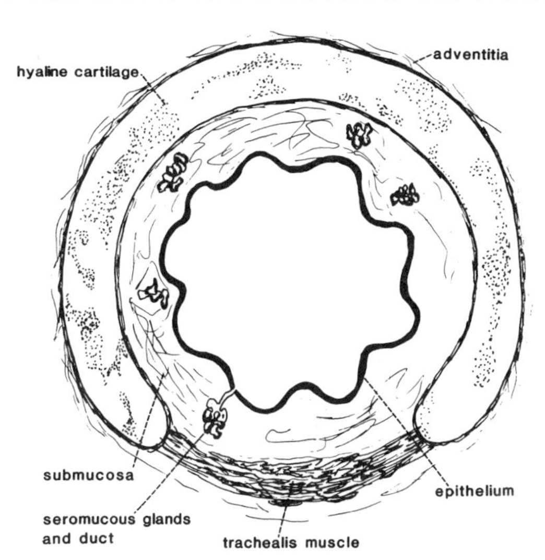


**Fig. 3.15.** Cross-section of the trachea.

rings are united by a band of smooth muscle cells, the trachealis muscle. The trachea branches into two mainstem or primary bronchi which, although somewhat smaller, mirror the features of the trachea. The trachea and bronchi are lined by pseudostratified ciliated columnar epithelium beneath which is located an unusually robust basement membrane, a submucosa containing loose connective tissue and seromucous glands and an adventitia of denser connective tissue. Goblet cells are numerous throughout the epithelium. Besides the more common ciliated cells and goblet cells which comprise the mucociliary apparatus for the removal of particulate material, a variety of other cells identifiable by electron microscopy may be present in the epithelium. These include:

1) Short or basal cells - rest on the basal lamina but do not reach the lumen. They are considered to be undifferentiated reserve (stem) cells.

2) Brush cells - these cells possess an apical border of straight, uniform microvilli rather than cilia. They are considered by some authorities to represent an inactive stage of the goblet cell and by others a type of sensory receptor cell.

3) Small granule cells - are located basally, usually do not reach the lumen, and contain small, dense-cored

granules. Some of these cells may produce catecholamines (neuroendocrine cells) while others produce protein hormones like those of certain enteroendocrine cells of the intestinal epithelium (argentaffin cells).

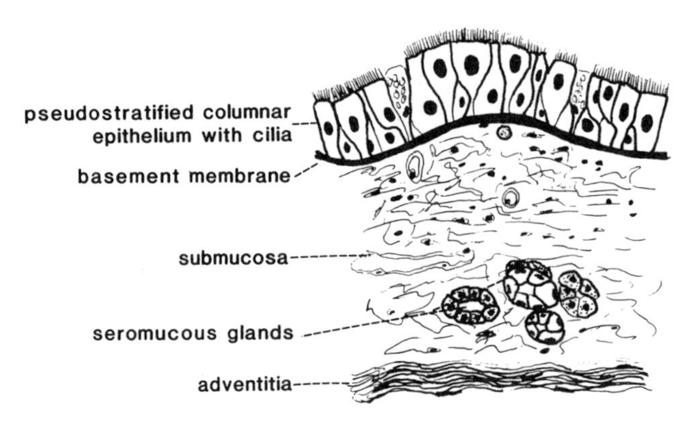


**Fig. 3.16.** Wall of a bronchus. between the cartilage plates.

Lungs, Intrapulmonary Bronchi and Bronchioles

The lungs are paired organs covered externally by a serous membrane (mesothelium + underlying connective tissue), the visceral pleura. The right and left mainstem (primary) bronchi and the pulmonary vessels (artery and veins) enter the lungs at the hilus. Each of the lobes (3 on the right, 2 on the left) receives a branch of the mainstem bronchus as a lobar (secondary) bronchus. Branches of the pulmonary arteries accompany the bronchial divisions. The lobar bronchi divide to eventually become segmental bronchi which supply the bronchopulmonary segments of each lobe (10 on the right, 8 on the left). An important anatomic feature of the bronchopulmonary segments is their relatively independent blood supply which makes surgical removal of one or more of these segments possible. The segmental bronchi continue to divide a number of times with a corresponding reduction in diameter and decrease in the amount of cartilage. As the cartilage decreases in amount, it becomes discontinuous so that it is represented by cartilaginous plates. Correspondingly, a spiraling layer of smooth muscle and elastic fibers, the muscularis mucosa, appears and increases in thickness as the cartilage is successively reduced. When the caliber is reduced to approximately 1 mm, the cartilage is absent and the term bronchiole is appropriate. Bronchioles continue to divide to the final, smallest form of the conducting division, the terminal bronchiole.

Bronchioles vary in size from about 1 mm to 0.3 mm. The walls of bronchioles in the conducting division lack (by definition) cartilaginous plates. The epithelium is simple columnar to cuboidal. Goblet cells disappear in the most distal segments but ciliated cells continue to be present. Scattered among the epithelial cells are nonciliated, dome-shaped secretory cells whose apices protrude into the lumen. These are variously referred to descriptively as bronchiolar secretory cells or eponymically as Clara cells. They contain a basally located RER, a supranuclear Golgi apparatus and apically located SER and numerous electron-dense secretory granules of a protein nature. Although their complete functional role is unclear, Clara cells are known to contribute surfactant to the bronchiolar fluid. Beneath the epithelium, a prominent layer of smooth muscle reinforced by elastic fibers is present. The terminal bronchioles are continuous with the respiratory bronchioles, the first segment of the respiratory division.

## Respiratory Division

The terminal bronchioles give rise to two orders of respiratory bronchioles. The structure of the respiratory bronchiole differs little from that of the terminal bronchiole with an important exception. Respiratory bronchioles possess alveoli which pouch outward from their walls and increase in number distally. It is only at the level of alveoli that the distance between blood and air becomes reduced to the point that gaseous exchange may occur. Thus the respiratory bronchiole is the first

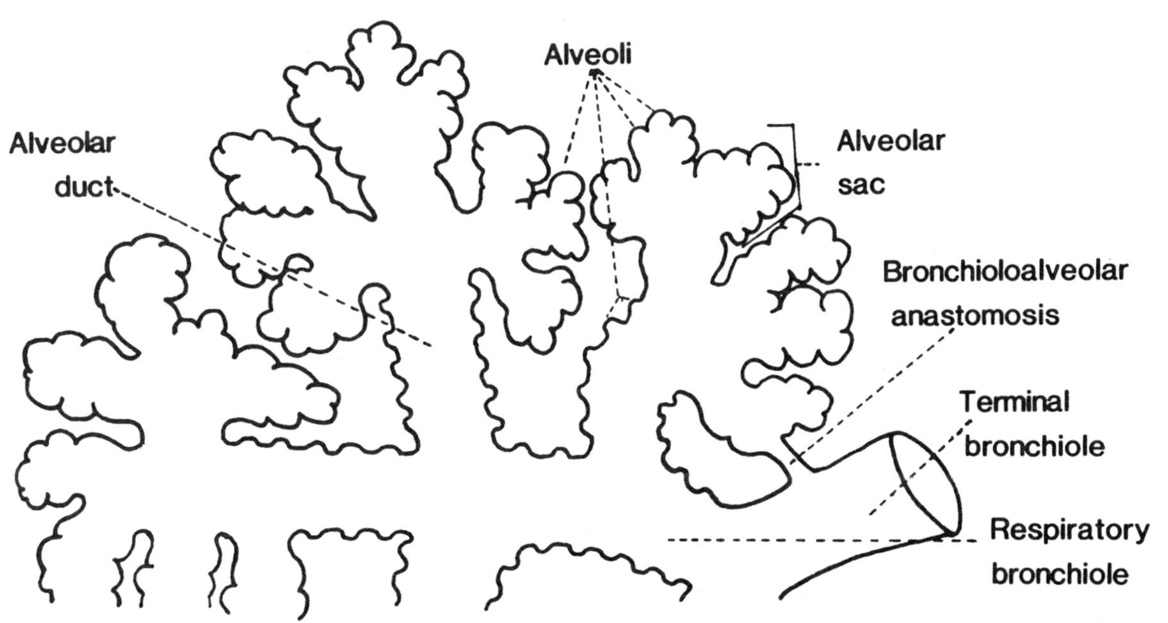


**Fig. 3.17.** Terminal bronchiole and respiratory division of the lung.

segment of the lung in which respiratory function occurs. It is not, however, the only portion and each successive structure is capable of gaseous exchange. Respiratory bronchioles give rise to alveolar ducts. These short segments have many alveoli associated with their walls and soon end in a number of alveolar sacs. Each alveolar sac consists of several to many alveoli which open into a common chamber, the atrium.

Alveoli are characterized by a polyhedral or polygonal shape with an opening on one aspect to permit the inflow of air from an adjacent respiratory bronchiole, alveolar duct or atrium. Because of the proximity of alveoli especially within the alveolar sacs, they often share walls with neighboring alveoli. This intervening structure is called an interalveolar septum. Occasionally, it may be penetrated by a small (7 to 15 microns) opening, the alveolar pore (of Kohn). These curious structures allow the equalization of pressure differences in adjacent alveoli especially of those originating from different bronchioles. They also allow collateral air flow to alveoli whose conducting bronchiole is obstructed.

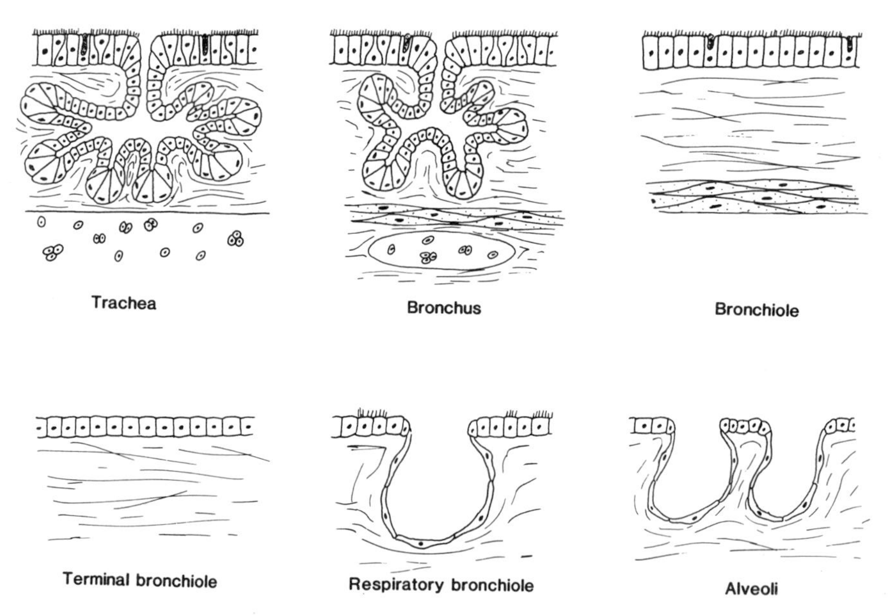


**Fig. 3.18.** Comparison of conducting and respiratory structures. (Courtesy Dr. R. Snell.)

The alveolar epithelium is physiologically important but structurally simple. It consists of a complete, highly attenuated squamous layer of epithelial cells termed Type I alveolar cells or Type I pneumocytes joined to each other by occluding (tight) junctions and occasional desmosomes. Between the Type I pneumocytes may be found single or small groups of another type of cell, termed variously, great alveolar cells, Type II alveolar cells, septal cells, granular pneumocytes or Type II pneumocytes. They are connected to the Type I pneumocytes by occluding junctions, are somewhat cuboidal or dome-shaped and may bulge into the alveolar spaces. They are commonly found at the corners or angles of alveolar walls. By light microscopy, they are characterized by a vacuolated cytoplasm. By EM, they contain conspicuous supranuclear collections of dense, multilamellar secretory granules. The secretory granules are precursors of a phospholipid-rich (75-85% phosphatidyl choline) surfactant. Within the interalveolar spaces and along the alveolar walls in the air spaces may be found an additional cell type, the pulmonary alveolar macrophage (PAM), of blood monocyte origin whose

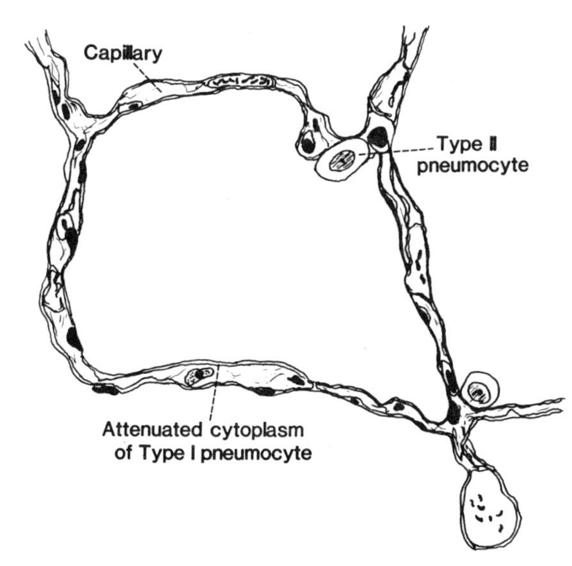


**Fig. 3.19.** The alveolus.

function is primarily one of phagocytosis and augmentation of B- and T-lymphocyte immune responses.

The lung has a rich network of continuous, nonfenestrated capillaries that occupy much of the space of the interalveolar septa. In regions where the Type I pneumocyte epithelium and the endothelium of the pulmonary capillaries are in close apposition, they may share a common basement membrane. It is across this tripartite structure (alveolar membrane, respiratory membrane) that gaseous exchange occurs. The three parts of the all important respiratory membrane include the attenuated cytoplasm of the Type I pneumocyte, the fused basement membranes and the cytoplasm of the endothelial cell.

# URINARY SYSTEM

The urinary system consists of the kidneys, ureters, urinary bladder and urethra. The functions of the kidney include elimination of waste metabolites (excretion), regulation of water and electrolyte balance (selective reabsorption and secretion) and the synthesis of renin and erythropoietin. The successive structures (ureters, urinary bladder and urethra) function to transport, temporarily store and eliminate urine.

## Kidney

The kidney is bean-shaped with an indentation (hilus) on the medial aspect at which the ureter and renal vein exit and the renal artery enters. Beneath the hilus is a cavity, the renal sinus, that contains the renal pelvis, a continuation of the ureter. The pelvis is subdivided into 2 or 3 major calyces from which branch several minor calyces (3 to 4 per major calyx or 8 to 12 total per kidney). The kidney is enclosed by a easily stripped fibroelastic capsule. The fact that it can be removed indicates that septae or trabeculae do not extend from it into the substance of the organ.

The kidney is composed of a cortex and medulla. The cortex contains both renal corpuscles and tubules. Within the medulla are several (6-12) medullary pyramids whose bases are oriented toward the cortex with conical apices (papillae) protruding into a minor calyx. The medullary pyramids have a striated appearance caused by a parallel arrangement of uriniferous tubules and blood vessels. Medullary substance extends from the bases of the medullary pyramids into the cortex as medullary rays. (NOTE: The medullary pyramids are part of the medulla; the medullary rays are part of the cortex.) The medullary pyramids are separated by downward extensions of cortical tissue, the renal columns (of Bertin). A renal lobe consists of a renal pyramid, the cortical tissue that surrounds it (renal columns) and the cortical tissue that overlies its base. Each lobe drains into a minor calyx at the papilla. The apex of the papilla is pierced by several collecting tubules (papillary ducts of Bellini) whose orifices open on the area cribrosa. A renal lobule consists of a medullary ray and the surrounding cortical tissue.

The pelvis, major and minor calyces are lined by a special epithelium peculiar to the urinary tract termed transitional epithelium or urothelium.

### Uriniferous Tubules

The uriniferous tubules comprise the nephrons which produce urine and the collecting tubules which function in conduction and hypertonic concentration of urine. Theses structures, although continuous, have a different developmental history.

The nephron is a blind-ended tubule whose most proximal portion is expanded. The blind saccular part comprises Bowman's capsule. It is indented by a capillary tuft of fenestrated glomerular capillaries. This structure (Bowman's capsule + capillary tuft) is termed the renal corpuscle. Renal corpuscles are confined to the cortex and are the site of plasma ultrafiltration. Fluid and certain molecular constituents of the plasma pass from the glomerular capillaries into the lumen of Bowman's capsule (Bowman's space). The glomerular ultrafiltrate then passes through segments of the nephron (where it is modified) to pass into the collecting tubule. Other segments of the nephron include (in order from Bowman's capsule): convoluted and straight portions of the proximal tubule, thin segment, straight and convoluted segment of distal tubule. Both proximal and distal convoluted segments are present within the cortex while the straight segments of both proximal and distal tubules as well as thin segments (which collectively comprise the loop of Henle) may extend downward into the medulla. In the cortex, a number of distal convoluted tubules empty into collecting ducts via short arched collecting tubules.

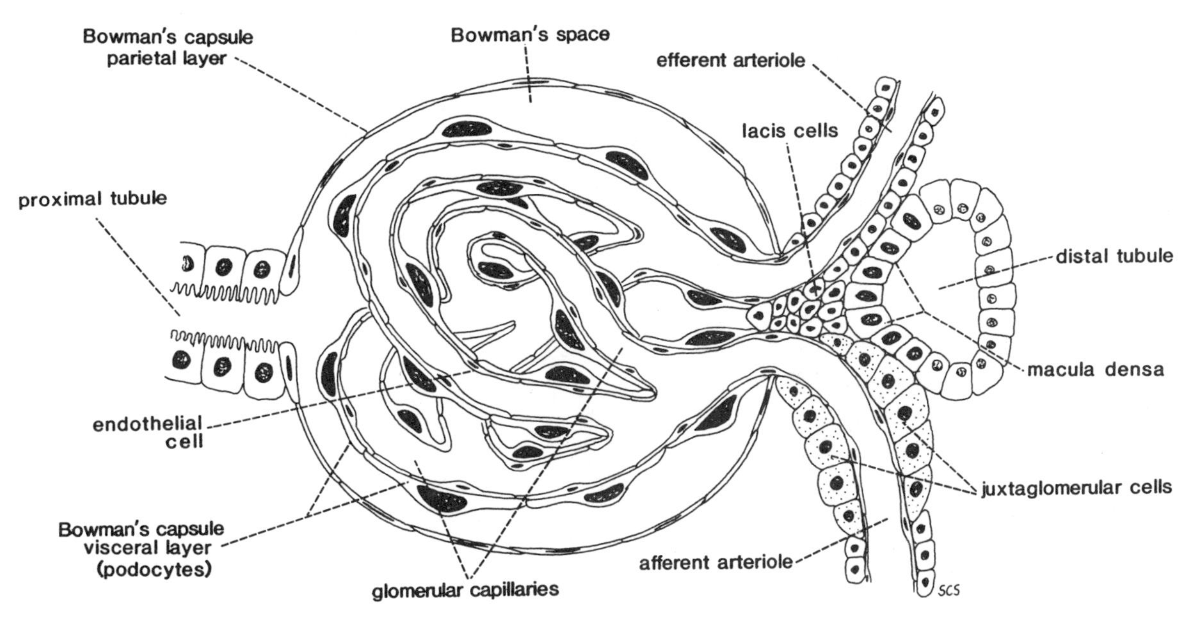


**Fig. 3.20.** The renal corpuscle and the juxtaglomerular apparatus.

The renal corpuscle contains a tubular pole where the parietal layer of Bowman's capsule is continuous with the proximal convoluted tubule and at the opposite end, a vascular pole where the afferent and efferent vessels (arterioles) that enter and leave the glomerulus are located. The parietal layer of Bowman's capsule is simple squamous epithelium that rests on a basal lamina located on the abluminal side of Bowman's space. The epithelium of Bowman's capsule reflects onto and covers the glomerular capillary tuft as the visceral layer. This epithelial layer is a structurally modified epithelium that functions as part of the filtration apparatus. The epithelial cells of the visceral layer of Bowman's capsule are stellate shaped cells called podocytes. Extending downward from the cell body toward the basal lamina that completely invests the glomerular capillaries are a number of (5-10) primary processes. The primary

GLOMERULAR ULTRASTRUCTURE

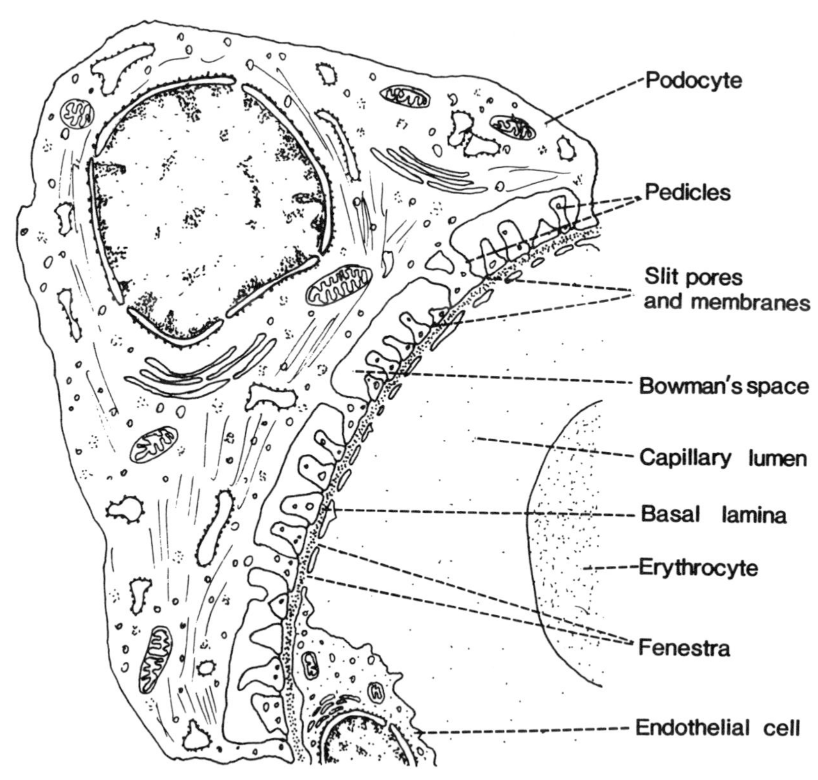


**Fig. 3.21.** Ultrastructure of the renal corpuscle.

processes branch into numerous secondary processes termed pedicles or foot processes. The pedicles rest directly on the basal lamina covering the fenestrated glomerular capillaries and interdigitate randomly with those from other podocytes to form a complete covering. Between adjacent pedicles are small spaces called slit pores or filtration slits. These are covered by a thin diaphragm or membrane. The slit diaphragms and the basal lamina together comprise the ultrastructural barrier across which all substances entering the urinary space (Bowman's space) from the glomerular capillaries must pass.

## KIDNEY TUBULES

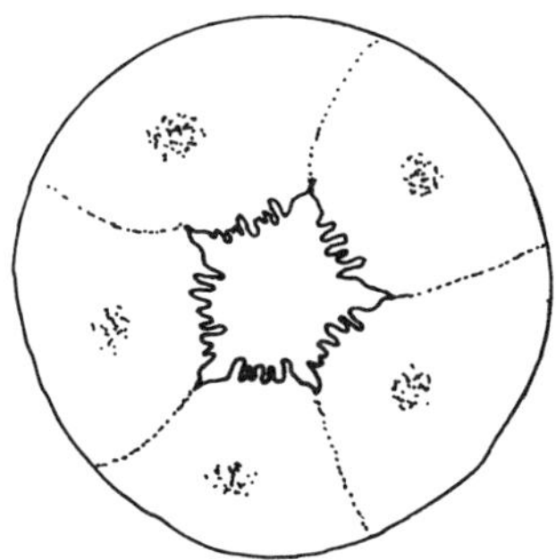
Proximal convoluted tubule

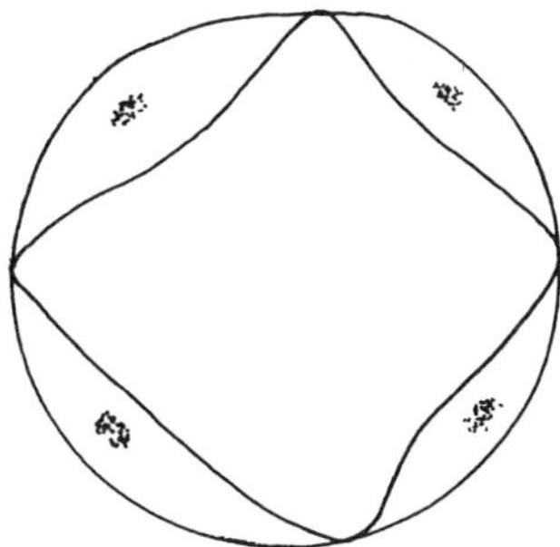
Loop of Henle (thin segment)

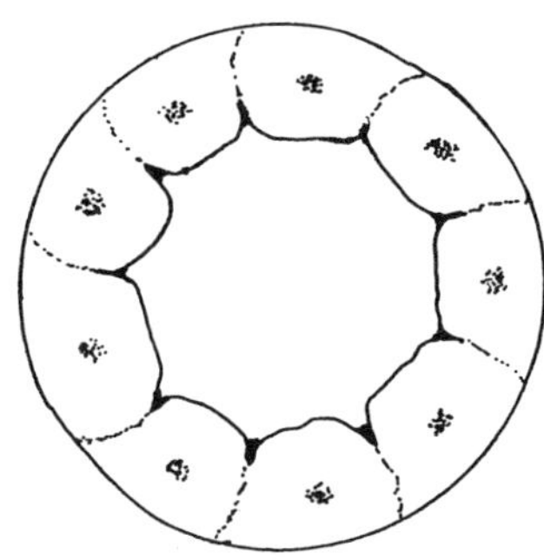
Distal convoluted tubule

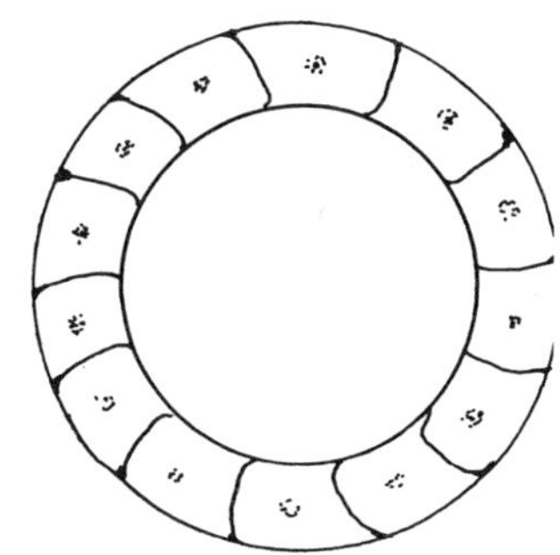
Collecting tubule

**Fig. 3.22.** Segments of tubules.

Both convoluted and straight segments of the proximal tubule cells are similar. They consist of a single layer of cuboidal cells that interdigitate laterally with their neighbors. On the apical surface are long microvilli constituting a brush border. Associated with the brush border is an extracellular glycocalyx that contains alkaline phosphatase and ATPase activity. This well-developed apical modification correlates with the chief function of the proximal tubules, the selective reabsorption of certain ions and molecules from the glomerular filtrate. Numerous long mitochondria are present in the basal cytoplasm.

The thin segments of the loop of Henle unite the straight portions of the proximal and distal tubules. The transition of the thick segments of the descending and ascending limbs into the thin segment occurs abruptly. The thin segments are lined by a few simple squamous epithelial cells whose nuclei tend to bulge into the lumen. Very few microvilli, not visible by light microscopy, are present on the apical surface. The cytoplasm contains only a few mitochondria and other organelles.

The distal tubule has a lumen that is larger than that of the proximal tubule. Fewer and shorter microvilli are present on the luminal surface and the cuboidal epithelial cells are shorter. Basal infoldings of the plasma membrane and associated longitudinally arranged mitochondria give the basal cytoplasm a striate appearance. This structural modification is associated with the active transport of ions (i.e., sodium cations).

The collecting tubules are not considered a component of the nephron but are the uriniferous tubules that transports and concentrates the urine. A number of distal tubules connect with the collecting tubule by way of short arched collecting tubules in the medullary rays. The collecting ducts traverse the length of the medullary rays to enter the medullary pyramids. Several collecting tubules join to form a single larger papillary duct. The cells forming the collecting tubules are cuboidal with distinct lateral and luminal cells boundaries. The epithelium gradually increases in height to become columnar at the level of papillary ducts. The collecting tubules are influenced by the action of antidiuretic hormone (ADH) which promotes water loss from the tubular fluid into the interstitium.

## Juxtaglomerular Apparatus

The juxtaglomerular apparatus (JGA) consists of a number of specialized cells. The function of the JGA is to regulate blood pressure by the production and timely release of the hormone renin. Renin acts on a circulating protein angiotensinogen to produce an inactive intermediary, angiotensin I. Angiotensin I is enzymatically activated in the lung to form angiotensin II, a potent vasoconstrictor peptide. Angiotensin II also stimulates secretion of aldosterone by the cells of the zona glomerulosa in the adrenal cortex. Aldosterone in turn promotes sodium and chloride ion resorption in the kidney and a subsequent increase in circulating blood volume. The components of the JGA include:

1) Juxtaglomerular (JG) cells - these are modified smooth muscle cells in the media of the afferent arteriole. Large cytoplasmic granules in these cells have been shown by immunocytochemistry to contain renin.

2) Macula densa - this is a nest of specialized cells in the wall of the distal convoluted tubule at the vascular pole of the renal corpuscle that are in direct physical contact with JG cells.

3) Lacis cells - these cells are extraglomerular mesangial

3) Lacis cells - these cells are extraglomerular mesangial cells located in the angle between the afferent and efferent arterioles at the vascular pole of the renal corpuscle. Their function is unclear but have been proposed to be the site of erythropoietin synthesis, a hormone known to be produced by the kidneys.

## Blood Supply

The renal artery enters at the hilus to divide into dorsal and ventral branches which split into several interlobar arteries. The interlobar arteries run in the cortical columns between the pyramids and ascend to the corticomedullary junction. At the junctional level, the interlobar arteries bifurcate into arcuate arteries that extend between the bases of the medullary pyramids and the overlying cortex. From these smaller interlobular arteries ascend into the cortex between the medullary rays where they give off the afferent arterioles that supply the cortical glomeruli. The efferent arterioles from the cortical and juxtamedullary glomeruli differ in their distribution. The chief difference is that the efferent arterioles of cortical glomeruli form a peritubular capillary plexus while the efferent arterioles of juxtamedullary glomeruli descend into the medulla as the vasa recta to eventually turn and ascend back into the cortex. The descending limbs of the vasa recta are termed the arteriolae rectae while the ascending limbs are called the venae rectae. Together they constitute the rete mirabile which function as countercurrent exchangers.

## Ureters, Urinary Bladder and Urethrae

The ureters are lined by transitional epithelium. The wall of the upper ureter contains a muscular coat consisting of an inner longitudinal and outer circular layer. (NOTE: this arrangement is opposite than that encountered in many other tubular structures.) In the lower segment (lower third) an additional outer longitudinal layer is present so that the circular layer now lies in the middle. Elastic fibers are abundant in the lamina propria between the epithelium and the muscular coat so that the empty ureter is characterized by longitudinal folds so that in cross section the lumen present a stellate appearance. The adventitia contains blood vessels, nerve trunks and ganglia.

The urinary bladder is also lined by urothelium that is somewhat thicker than that of the ureter. The muscular wall consists of the same three coats as the lower ureter. The middle circular layer functions in the area of the internal urethral opening as a sphincter. Adventitia covers all but the dome which is surfaced by the pelvic peritoneum.

The urethral lining is variable in both males and females. Patches of pseudostatified or stratified columar as well as stratified squamous may be encountered.

## DIGESTIVE SYSTEM

The digestive system begins with the oral cavity and continues to the anus as a tubular organ along which various structural and functional modifications occur. Associated with the oral cavity and digestive tube are various accessory organs which function in the digestive process. These include the salivary glands, pancreas and liver.

### Oral Cavity

The buccal cavity and oropharynx are covered by a moist stratified squamous epithelium.

The teeth are hard organs which function in mastication. There are 20 deciduous teeth that are subsequently replaced by the 32 permanent teeth. Although the shape of various teeth (incisures, molars) differs, their basic structure is similar. The central portion of teeth (pulp chamber) contains the dental pulp, a loose connective tissue containing nerves and vessels which enter at the apical foramen. The dental pulp is surrounded by a single layer of odontoblasts. These cells secrete the next layer of predentin. A deeper layer secreted previously has undergone mineralization and is termed dentin. Dentin is approximately 69% mineral. Long, slender cytoplasmic processes (Tome's fibers) of the odontoblasts extend throughout the thickness of the dentin within minute canals, the dentinal tubules. During development of the teeth, the odontoblasts induce an ectodermally derived layer of cells, the ameloblasts, to secrete the outer layer of enamel which covers the exposed portions of erupted teeth. Enamel is acellular, totally nonvital and is greater than 96% inorganic material. The ameloblastic epithelium is absent from erupted teeth. Covering the root of the tooth is another mineralized substance, similar to bone but avascular, known as cementum. It is secreted by cells called cementocytes which like osteocytes become entrapped in their mineralized extracellular matrix. The root of the tooth is firmly anchored into the surrounding alveolar bone by the fibrous periodontal ligament (PDL).

The tongue functions in mastication and speech. Its main mass is skeletal muscle whose fibers diverge in many directions. The tongue is surfaced by a stratified squamous epithelium. On the dorsum are found three types of papillae, the filiform, fungiform and circumvallate. Taste buds are associated with the latter two types.

### General Features of Tubular Viscera

The tubular viscera of the digestive system possess certain common features. Although occasional variations to the basic plan occur it is convenient to recall first the common structural

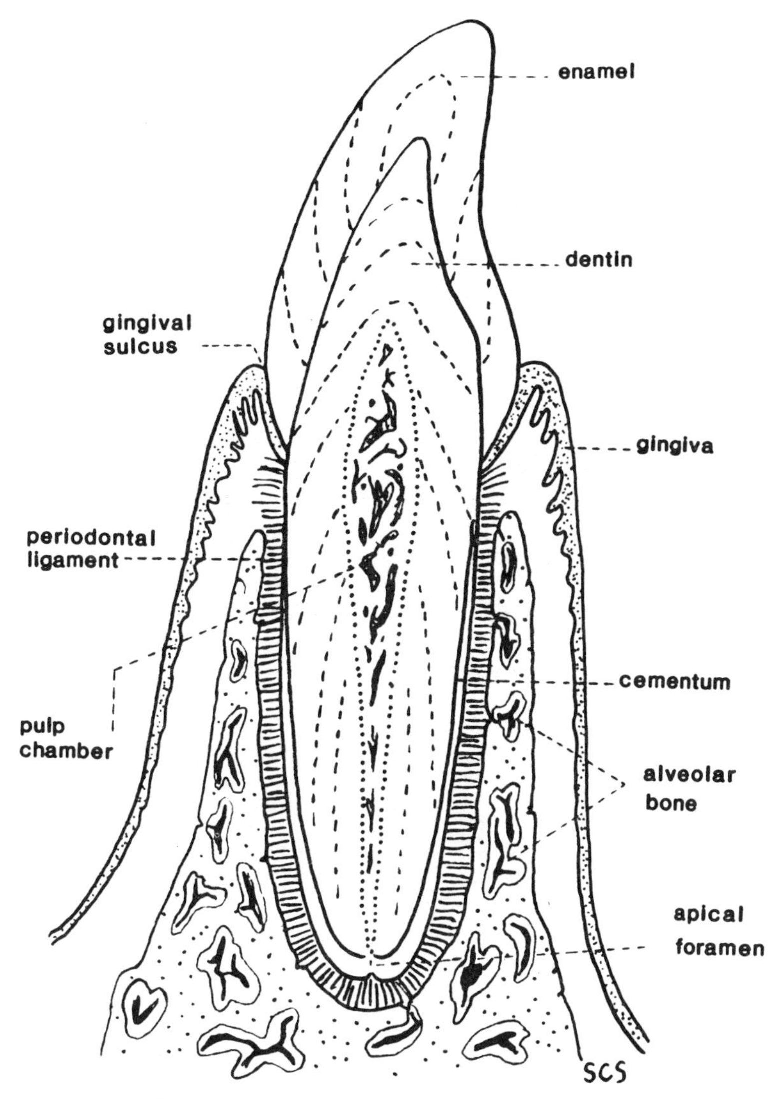


**Fig. 3.23.** Diagrammatic representation of a tooth.

features and then address the exceptions as they arise. The four main layers from the lumen to the outside include a mucosa, submucosa, muscularis externa and adventitia (or serosa).

The mucosa consists of four layers. In order from the lumen outward these are the epithelium, basement membrane, lamina propria and muscularis mucosae.

The submucosa lies between the muscularis mucosae and the muscularis externa. It consists of a fairly loose connective tissue (areolar) which in some regions may contain glands (submucosal glands).

The muscularis externa consists of two or more layers of

muscle tissue which, depending on location, may be smooth muscle or smooth and skeletal muscle.

The adventitia is the outermost layer. If covered externally by mesothelium, the term serosa is appropriate.

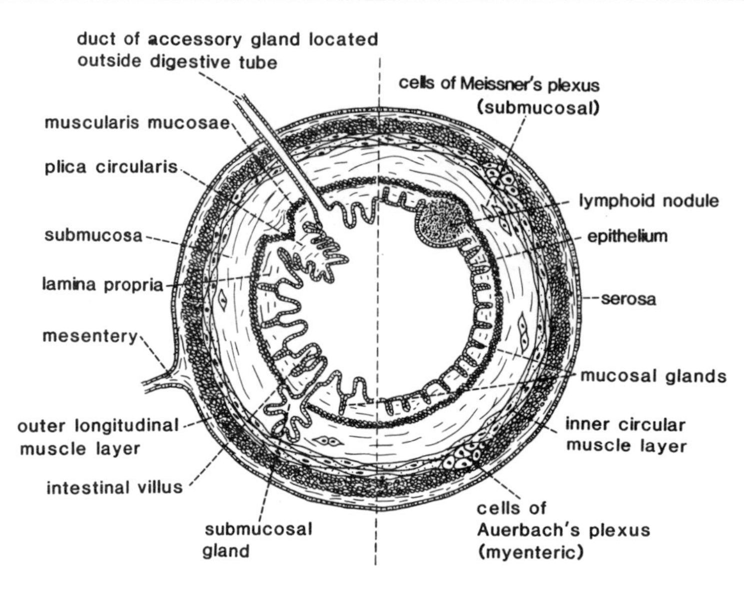


**Fig. 3.24.** Chief characteristics of the various regions of the digestive tube in a single composite drawing.

## Esophagus

The epithelium of the mucosa is a thick layer of moist stratified squamous. Small, mucous glands may be present in the mucosa (subsurface glands) and in the underlying submucosa. The muscularis mucosae is well-developed below the level of the cricoid cartilage and consists of a layer of longitudinally arranged smooth muscle cells. The submucosa contains longitudinally arranged collagenous and elastic fibers resulting in longitudinal folds in the mucosa which keep the lumen closed when empty. The muscularis externa consists of skeletal muscle fibers only in the upper third, a mixture of skeletal muscle and smooth muscle cells in the middle third and in the lower third, an inner circular and outer longitudinal arrangement of smooth muscle layers. This latter pattern is repeated throughout much of the rest of the digestive tube with minor alterations. The supradiaphragmatic esophagus is covered externally by an adventitia while below the diaphragm, a serosa is present.

## Stomach

The stomach is an expanded portion of the digestive tube

that serves as a tempory storage depot for food and is important in the initial stages of digestion. It secretes acid (HCl) and pepsinogen. The secretions and the muscular action of the stomach convert the food into a semisolid material known as chyme. Chyme is then passed into the small intestine where the bulk of digestion and absorption occur.

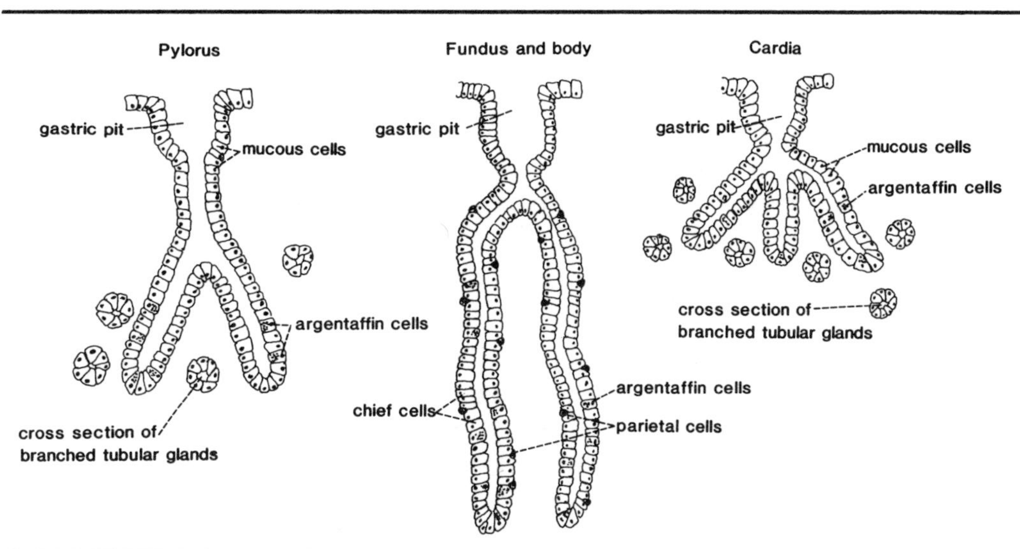


**Fig. 3.25.** Glands of the stomach regions. (Courtesy Dr. R. Snell)

## Mucosa

The mucosa of the stomach begins abruptly at the gastroesophageal junction to become simple columnar. It is quite thick due to numerous gastric glands that open onto the surface by way of gastric pits or foveolae. The glands vary in the different regions of the stomach.

The pyloric glands of the distal stomach are short, wide and coiled and of the simple, branching tubular type. The most common cell type in the pyloric glands are mucous-secreting cells among which are scattered a few so-called argentaffin cells.

The glands of the fundus and body (gastric glands) occupy the largest area and produce the bulk of the acid and enzymes of the gastric secretions. Cells include the parietal, chief, mucous neck and argentaffin to be discussed subsequently. The gastric pits are short and the glands are simple branched tubular whose secretory portions are long and straight.

The cardiac glands contain relatively shallow gastric pits. Most of the cells are mucous cells with only scattered argentaffin cells. The glands are simple coiled tubular or branched tubular in form.

The lamina propria is scanty in all these regions and extends between the glands which are located there. The muscularis mucosae is thin but arranged into visible layers. An inner circular layer, an outer longitudinal layer and occasionally a third external oblique layer may be discerned.

Epithelial Cells of the Gastric Mucosa

1) Surface epithelial cells - simple columnar epithelial cells that secrete mucous line the entire surface of the stomach (mucous secreting sheet). They also dip into the gastric pits. These cells produce a neutral mucous.

2) Mucous neck cells - present as single cells and in small groups in the necks of the gastric glands (fundus and body). They differ from surface mucous cells in that they are more irregular in shape and produce an acid mucous.

3) Chief (zymogenic) cells - found in the bases of the gastric glands. Cytoplasm is basophilic and contains a basally located, spherical nucleus, supranuclear Golgi apparatus and apical acidophilic zymogen granules. Chief cells secrete pepsinogen which is activated in the acid pH of the stomach to pepsin.

4) Parietal (oxyntic) cells - most numerous in upper portions of gastric glands where they occur singularly or in small groups. A few may be present in the cardiac and pyloric glands as well. Contain an acidophilic cytoplasm, a centrally positioned nucleus along which a laterally or basally located Golgi apparatus may be seen. Numerous mitochondria with prominent crista are present within the cytoplasm. The major and unique ultrastructural feature is the presence of so-called intracellular canaliculi. These appear as deep invaginations of the luminal surface from which project numerous microvillous processes. This increased luminal membrane surface area is functionally related to the major role of the parietal cell, the secretion of hydrochloric acid. Intrinsic factor is believed to be secreted by some parietal cells.

5) Argentaffin (enterochromaffin) cells - more recently termed enteroendocrine cells, they actually represent a composite of many different cells that in common secrete one of many different types of low molecular weight polypeptide hormones into the blood. Besides their common ability to stain with dichromate salts or silver methods, they contain basally located (sub-nuclear) granules. Depending on the peptide secreted, the cells may be subclassified. Gastrin or G cells are

located in the pyloric antrum and secrete gastrin which stimulates acid secretion by parietal cells and motility of the distal stomach. I cells are present in the stomach and small intestines where they secrete cholecystokinin which stimulates pancreatic acinar cell secretion and release of bile from the gallbladder. S cells of the distal stomach and proximal small bowel produce secretin that induces pancreatic release of an alkaline secretion. EC cells secrete serotonin and endorphins while ECL cells are thought to release histamine.

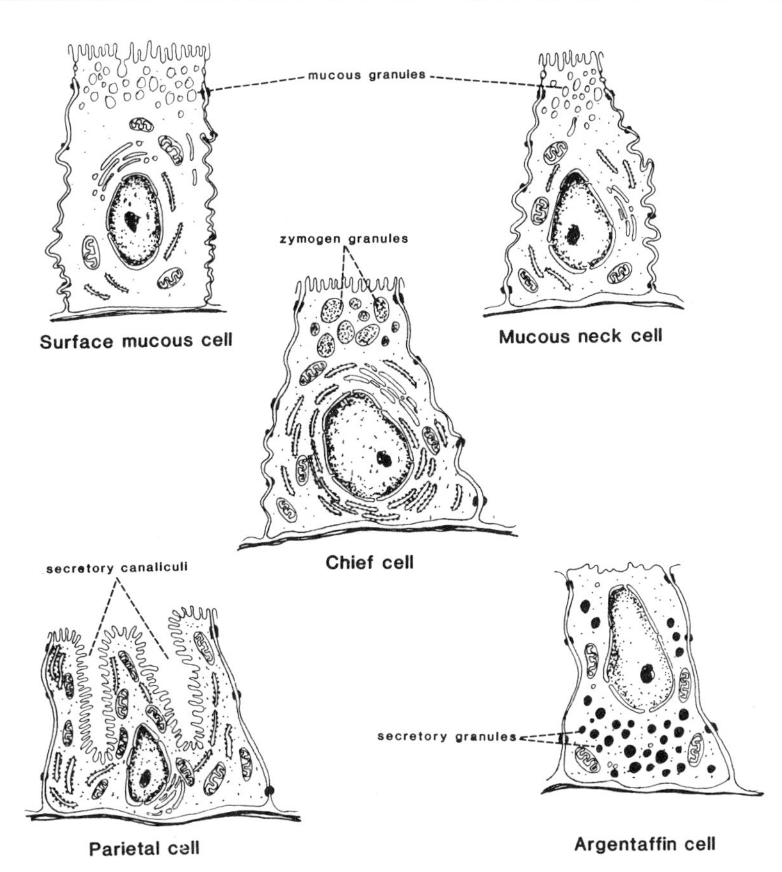


**Fig. 3.26.** Ultrastructure of gastric epithelial cells. (Courtesy Dr. R. Snell)

## Other Layers of the Stomach

1) Submucosa - loose connective tissue with collagen and elastic fibers that extends into and forms the rugae.

2) Muscularis externa - an outer longitudinal and middle circular layer are continuous with the two smooth

muscle layers of the lower esophagus. An additional irregular, inner oblique layer may be discerned.

3) Serosa - at the greater and lesser curvatures, a serosa is continuous with the greater and lesser omenta, respectively.

## Small Intestine

Extends from the pyloric region of the stomach to the ileocecal junction. Divided into duodenum, jejunum and ileum.

### Mucosa

The intestinal epithelium consists of a layer of simple columnar cells. Finger-like surface projections of the mucosa (villi) and subsurface invaginations (intestinal glands or crypts of Lieberkuhn) substantially increase the surface area of the intestines for absorption and secretion. Intestinal glands are present in both the small and large bowel but villi are restricted to the small intestine. The majority of cells (absorptive cells) covering the villi contain a prominent brush border of microvilli coated by a thick glycocalyx. Terminal bars are particularly prominent by light microscopy. Interspersed among the absorptive cells are mucous-secreting goblet cells. The glands contain occasional argentaffin cells and in the base of each crypt, groups of Paneth cells with acidophilic apical cytoplasmic granules. These cells are known to secrete lysozyme but their complete functional role is unclear. All of the intestinal cells are joined together at their lateral borders by junction complexes.

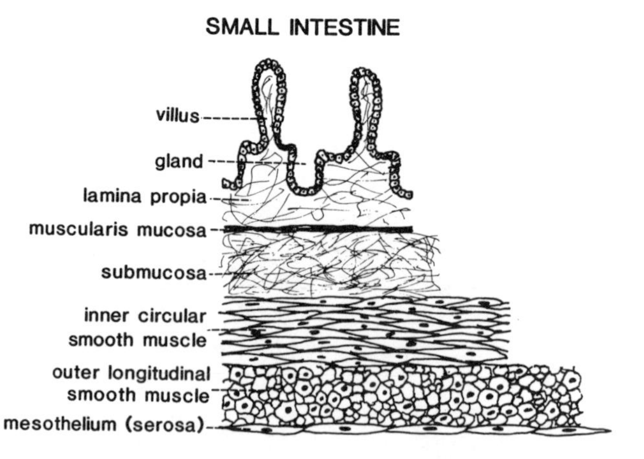


**Fig. 3.27.** Cross section of small intestinal wall. (Courtesy Dr. R. Snell)

## Other Layers of the Small Intestine

Below the epithelial basement membrane is the lamina propria that extends into each villus and surrounds each crypt. Present in the lamina propria of villi is a blood capillary plexus and the blind saccular or looped beginning of a lymphatic capillary known as the lacteal of the villus. Lymphoid nodules may be present throughout the small intestine but may be particularly prominent as aggregates in the ileum (Peyer's patches). They always occur on the side of the gut opposite the mesenteric attachment. A conspicuous muscularis mucosae lies beneath the lamina propria.

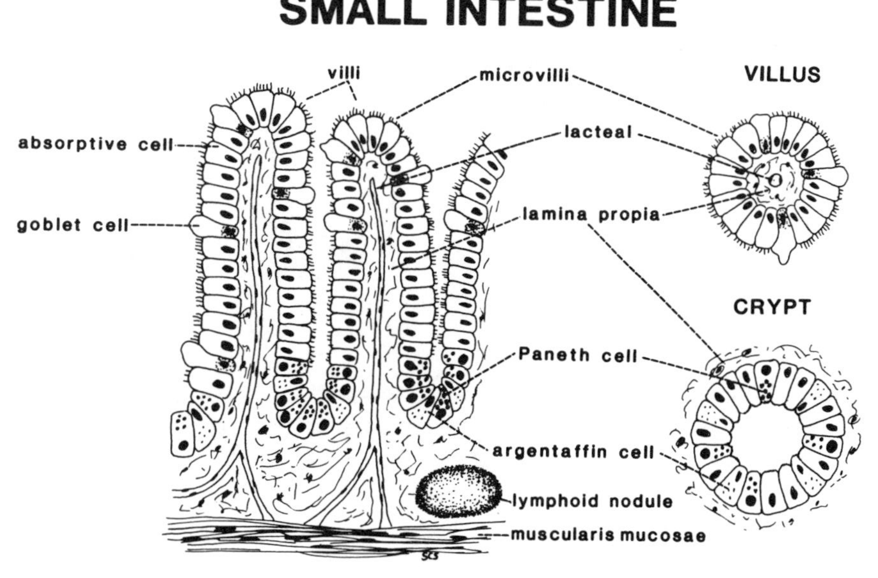


**Fig. 3.28.** Mucosa of the small intestine.

The submucosa is fairly nondescript except in the duodenum where a thick layer of submucosal glands (of Brunner) are located. The muscularis mucosae overlying these glands is often deficient. They secrete an alkaline mucous into the intestinal lumen that protects the proximal small intestine from the acidic gastric contents as they pass into it. Ganglion cells and nerves of Meissner's plexus are present within the submucosa. (Remember: Meissner's/subMucosa).

The muscularis externa consists of an inner circular and outer longitudinal layer of smooth muscle. Between the two layers are ganglion cells of Auerbach's myenteric plexus. (Remember: Auerbach's Myenteric/Muscularis externa). Most of the small intestine is covered externally on at least some aspects by a serosa. Retroperitoneal segments are covered by adventitia.

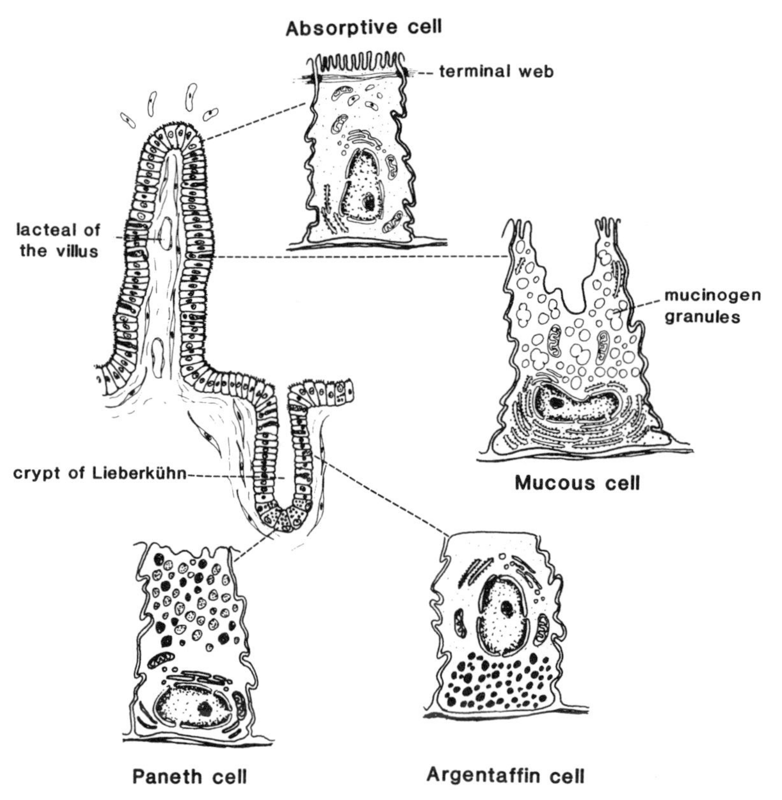


**Fig. 3.29.** Ultrastructure of intestinal cells. (Courtesy Dr. R. Snell)

## Large Intestine

The surface epithelium is simple columnar. Villi are not present and the subsurface glands (crypts of Lieberkuhn) are simple tubular and straight. Many of the cells are mucous-secreting mixed with occasional absorptive cells with apical microvilli. The mucous cells increase in density distally while the Paneth cells become less common. The laminal propria may contain lymphoid nodules which bulge into the submucosa. A well-developed muscularis mucosae is discernable. The inner circular layer of the muscularis externa is complete but the outer longitudinal layer is present as three narrow bands, the taeniae coli. A serosa covers the bulk of the colon especially the transverse segment but is not associated with portions of the ascending and descending segments. When present, the serosa may contain grossly visible fatty tissue, the appendices epiploicae.

## Appendix

The appendix is a thin, blind diverticulum of the cecum.

The surface epithelium contains only a few goblet cells and the crypt epithelium may contain both argentaffin and a few Paneth cells. The small, central lumen is often thrown into deep folds. The lamina propria is conspicuous because of the large numbers of lymphoid nodules that occupy it. They often extend through the muscularis mucosae into the relatively thick submucosa which contains numerous fat cells. The rest of the wall consists of a typical two-layered muscularis externa and is covered externally by a serosa.

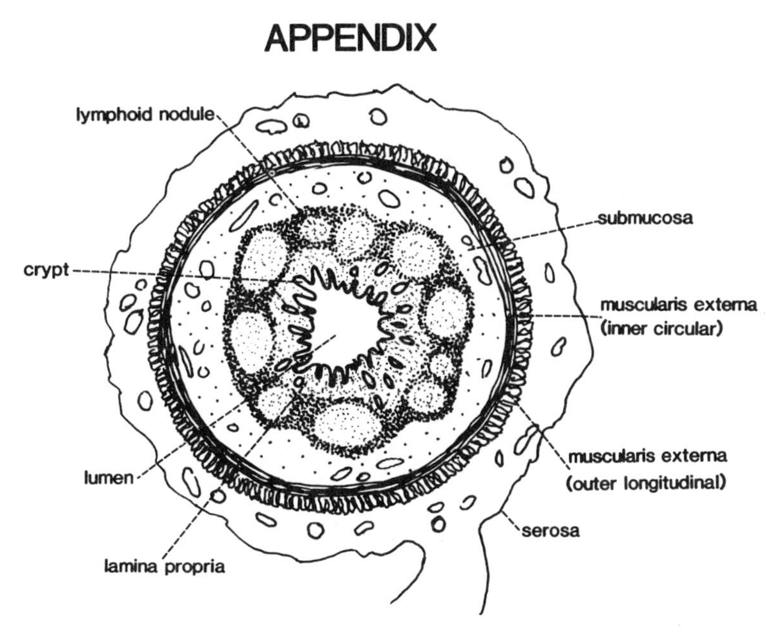


**Fig. 3.30.** Structure of the appendix.

## Accessory Organs of the Digestive System

The accessory organs are glands. Associated with the oral cavity are the major salivary glands that secrete salivary amylase and mucous. The pancreas (exocrine portion) and liver are associated with the small intestine. Ducts connect the extramural accessory glands with their respective portions of the digestive tube.

### Major Salivary Glands

The secretions of the major salivary glands (parotids, submandibular and sublinguals) pass into the oral cavity via ducts. Ducts within the glands begin as intralobular ducts that are quite thin and often branched. These narrow ductal segments are known as intercalated ducts. They are continuous with the next larger order of intralobular ducts lined by ductal cells bearing prominent basal striations. These are termed striated ducts and function in ionic and water transport. Striated ducts connect with larger interlobular ducts which drain into the primary duct. The secretory product of each gland can be predicted by the structure of the type(s) of secretory acini. Depending on the specific gland, serous, mucous, seromucous acini or combinations of the above may be present.

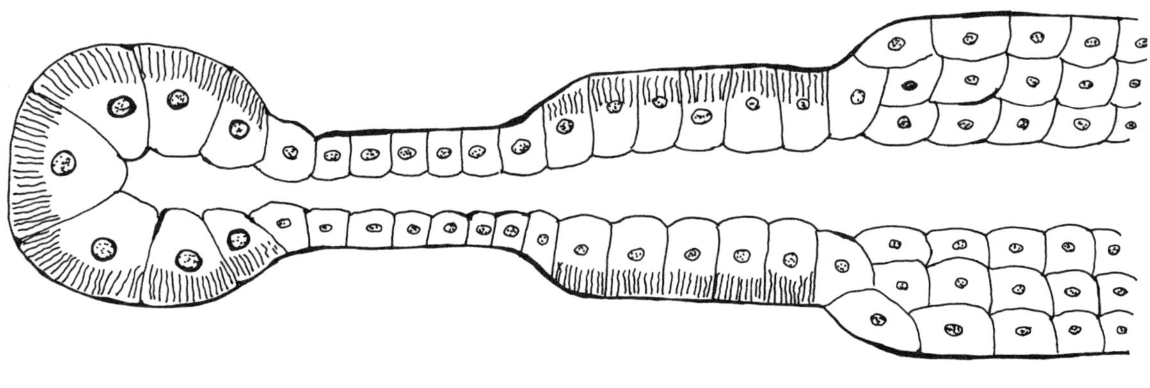


**Fig. 3.31.** Diagramatic representation of a salivary gland duct.

1) Parotid gland - largest of the salivary glands, it main duct is called Stensen's duct. Secretory acini are invariably serous. Long intercalated ducts and larger striated ducts are present. Myoepithelial cells are often present.

2) Submandibular gland - its main duct is termed Wharton's duct. Like the parotid, it is a compound tubuloalveolar gland. Although serous acini predominate, occasional mucous and seromucous acini are present. Less conspicuous and shorter intercalated but more prominent striated ducts are found.

3) Sublingual gland - a compound mixed tubuloalveolar gland in which the majority of acini are mucous. Occasional mucous acini capped externally by serous cells (serous demilunes) are found. Shorter and less conspicuous intercalated ducts are sparse or even absent. Striated ducts are present but rare.

## Pancreas

The pancreas consists of both an exocrine (acinar) and endocrine (islets of Langerhans) component.

The exocrine pancreas is composed of numerous acini or alveoli of 5 to 8 pyramidal cells disposed about a small (microscopic) central lumen. Pale-staining central cells (centroacinar cells) comprise the initial segments of the ductal system. The acinar cells contain a spherical, somewhat basally located nucleus bearing one or more prominent nucleoli. Their cytoplasm is basophilic in the basal portion where abundant RER and free ribosomes are located and more eosinophilic in the apical region due to the content of numerous zymogen granules. Secretory products include trypsin, chymotrypsin, carboxypeptidases, amylases and lipases as well as others. The intralobular ducts contain long, branched intercalated segments but lack striated portions. Interlobular ducts connect with either the main duct (of Wirsung) or the accessory duct (of Santorini).

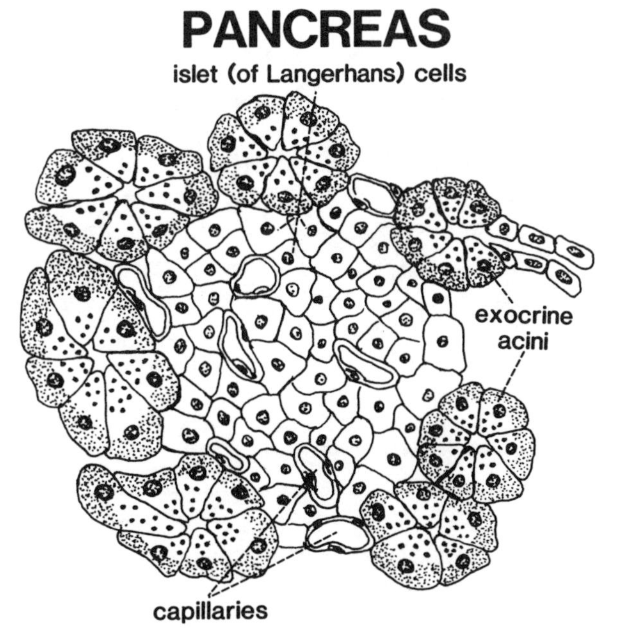

PANCREAS

islet (of Langerhans) cells

exocrine acini

capillaries

**Fig. 3.32.** Pancreatic islet and surrounding acini.

The endocrine pancreas is diffusely distributed throughout the pancreas as small groups of pale-staining cells that comprise the islets of Langerhans. Various cells types are present in the islets. The more common ones include:

1) A (alpha) cells - contain secretory vesicles with electron-dense cores. They release glucagon in

response to low blood glucose levels.

2) B (beta) cells - are the most numerous cell type (75%). Their zymogen granules contain a peculiar crystalloid core. The cells synthesize preinsulin which is converted into insulin and C-peptide in the Golgi apparatus before release.

3) C (clear) cells - are sparse, lack granules and of unknown function. They may be reserve cells.

4) D (delta) cells - contain variably sized granules and secrete somatostatin. A variant possessing smaller granules, the $D_1$ cell, secretes vasoactive intestinal peptide (VIP).

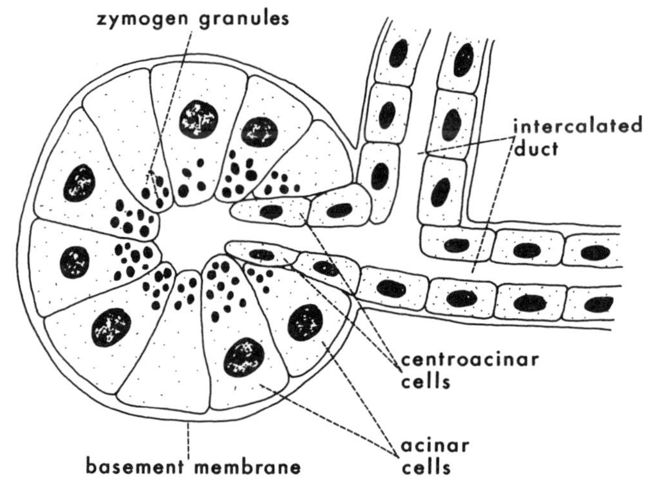


**Fig. 3.33.** Pancreatic acinus and intercalated duct.

## Liver and Gallbladder

The liver receives arterial blood from branches of the celiac trunk but the bulk of blood entering the liver is from the portal vein which carries material absorbed from the intestinal tract. The liver uses these absorbed materials to assimilate and store various substances. It is also important in the detoxification of various substances and excretes bile which is stored and concentrated by the gallbladder. Ducts from the liver and gallbladder eventually connect with the small intestine where they deliver bile salts that are important in fat digestion.

The parenchymal cells of the liver are epithelial cells of

endodermal origin termed hepatocytes. Hepatocytes are arranged in anastomosing and branching cords or plates. Between the cords are sinusoidal blood spaces lined by discontinuous endothelial cells. Characteristic lobules are present, delineated by peripherally placed portal areas. These are also termed portal triads because three characteristic structures are present.

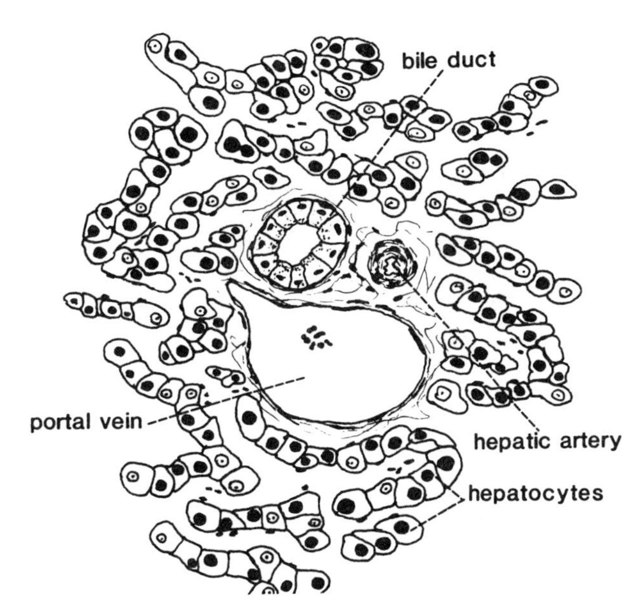


**Fig. 3.34.** The portal triad.

These include a branch of the hepatic artery, a branch of the portal vein and a small bile duct. Lymph vessels although not usually visualized by light microscopy are usually present as well. All of these structures are bound by small amounts of fibroconnective tissue.

The classical hepatic lobule has several peripherally arranged portal triads and a single central vein (venule) which represents a tributary of the inferior vena cava. The hepatocyte plates radiate outward from the central venule toward the portal areas. Blood flows from the afferent vessels, the portal vein and hepatic artery, toward the central vein through the sinusoidal spaces. Along the sinusoids are interposed occasional phagocytic cells (of Kupffer). By EM, a narrow space (of Disse) separates the sinusoidal endothelial cells from the underlying hepatocytes.

Bile secreted by the hepatocytes flows in small interhepatocytic channels, the bile canaliculi. At the EM level, the walls of canaliculi are seen to be composed of invaginations of adjacent hepatocyte plasma membrane from which microvilli protrude to enter the canalicular lumen. Intercellular junctions seal the edges of the canaliculi along their course. Bile formed in the hepatocytes flows passively through the canaliculi in the direction opposite of blood flow and connects abruptly with bile ducts in the portal triad via a small canal of Herring.

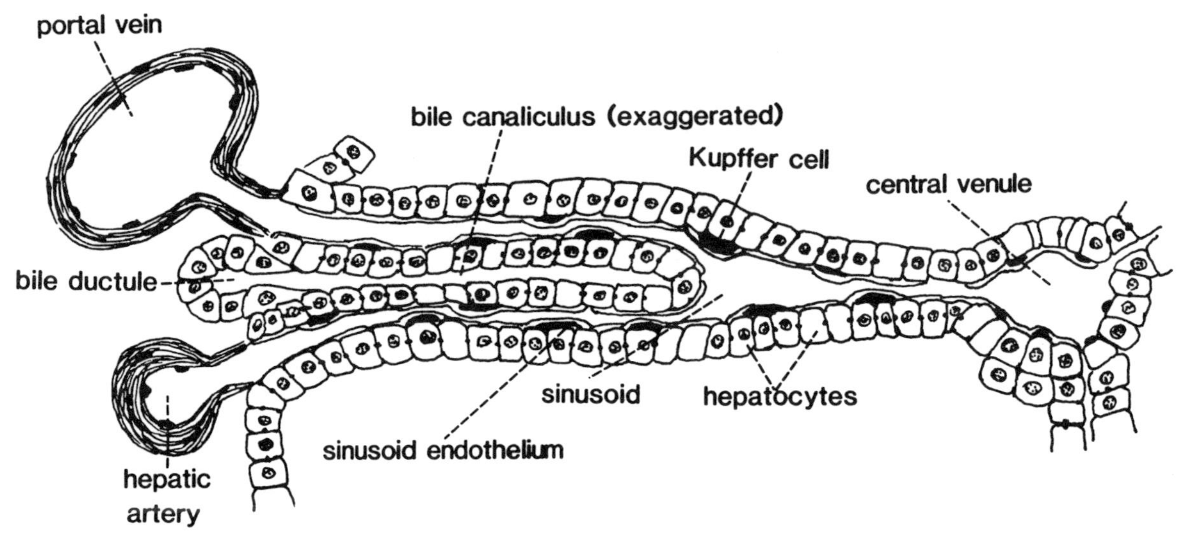


Fig. 3.35. Diagram of the classic liver lobule.

The hepatocyte nuclei are often large and polyploid and occasional binucleate cells are observed. The nuclei tend to be

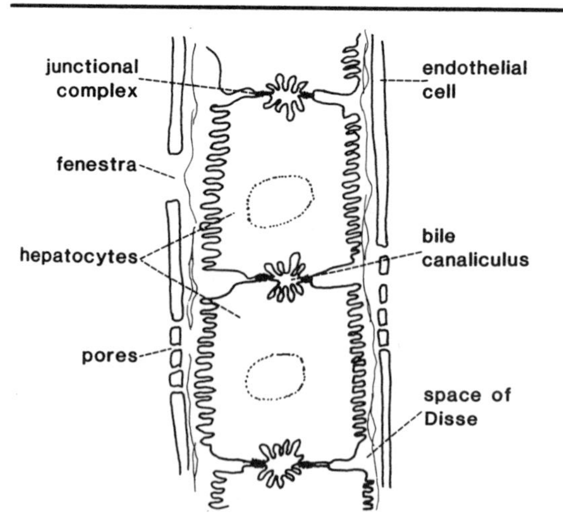


**Fig. 3.36.** Bile canaliculi and space of Disse.

vesicular and contain one or more nucleoli. The cytoplasmic borders tend to be well-defined and the cytoplasm itself is usually filled with clumps of basophilic material. Mitochondria are particularly abundant and representatives of the usual cellular organelles are present.

The gallbladder is a thin-walled blind diverticulum of the proximal common hepatic duct. Its wall is composed of a mucous membrane, a muscularis and an adventitia or serosa. The mucous membrane is thrown up into irregular folds. It is covered by a layer of simple columnar epithelial cells that may show apical microvilli. The muscularis is composed of irregularly oriented bundles of smooth muscle. The hepatic aspect of the gallbladder is covered by an adventitia, elsewhere it is covered by a serosa.

# MALE REPRODUCTIVE SYSTEM

The male reproductive system consists of the primary sex organs (the testes) and a successive series of excretory ducts along which are interposed a number of secondary sex organs. The testis produces the mature male germ cells (spermatozoa) and certain androgenic hormones responsible for various male characteristics. The secondary or accessory sex organs produce the fluid component of semen. These glandular structures include the seminal vesicles, prostate and bulbourethral (Cowper's) glands. During ejaculation, the excretory ductal system transports the cellular product of the testes (sperm) and the fluid media produced by the accessory glands. Components of the ductal system include tubuli recti, rete testis, efferent ductules, epididymis, vas deferens, ejaculatory duct and urethra. The urethra serves an additional role in the transport of urine from the urinary bladder during micturition. The male copulatory organ is the penis.

TESTIS AND EPIDIDYMIS

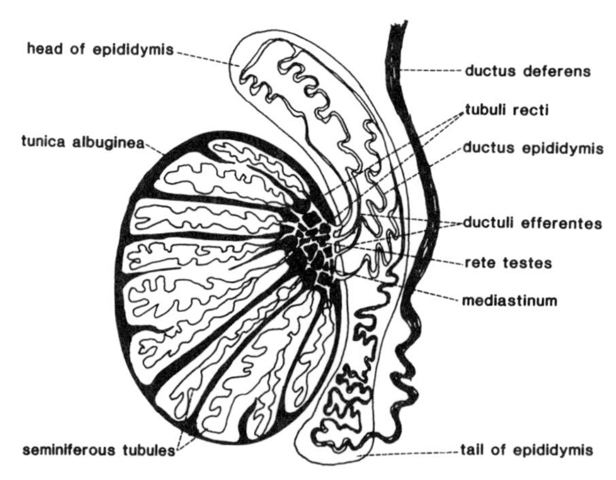


**Fig. 3.37.** Testis and its ducts

## Testes

The testis functions as both an exocrine and endocrine gland. Its exocrine product is in the form of mature sperm cells produced by proliferation and maturation of spermatogonia within the seminiferous tubules. Its endocrine product is in the form of androgenic steroid hormones produced by the interstitial (Leydig) cells located between the seminiferous tubules.

The major parenchymal component of the testis is the

seminiferous tubules. These highly convoluted tubules are lined by the germinal or seminiferous epithelium. In the mature, functional testis the seminiferous epithelium consists of a stratified layer of spermatogenic cells in various stages of differentiation and an interposed single layer of supporting (Sertoli) cells. Each individual Sertoli cell rests on the basal lamina and extends to the tubular lumen. They do not proliferate and unlike the spermatogenic cells are not of primordial germ cell origin. After onset of puberty, the spermatogenic cells proliferate constantly. Thus they belong to the constantly renewing or labile cell population. Because the mature cells (spermatozoa) are constantly being shed from the epithelial surface into the lumen of the seminiferous tubules, cells in the layers below consist of stem cells, proliferating cells and differentiating cells.

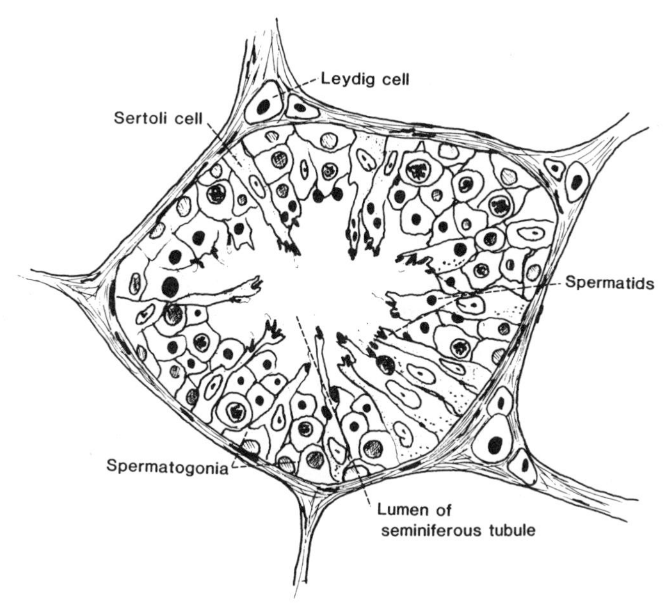


**Fig. 3.38.** Seminiferous tubule and interstitium.

Besides the Sertoli cells, the basal layer of cells includes special stem cells termed spermatogonia. There are three types based upon the morphology and staining characteristics of their nuclei. Two kinds of Type A spermatogonia are recognized. Both have ovoid nuclei but in one (pale Type A) the nucleus stains lightly and in the other it appears more deeply stained (dark Type A). The nucleus of the third type of spermatogonia (Type B) is round and marked by dark, punctate patches of heterochromatin. Dark Type A cells divide infrequently and function as reserve stem cells. Pale Type A cells divide by mitosis to produce more Type B cells and both types of A cells thereby maintaining the population of stem cells. The Type B cells divide mitotically and certain numbers of the daughter cells become primary spermatocytes. Primary spermatocytes then enter the first meiotic division to become secondary spermatocytes which in turn enter the second meiotic division to become haploid spermatids. Through a process of morphogenesis known as spermiogenesis the spermatids differentiate into mature, functional spermatozoa.

The function of the Sertoli cells as a supporting element is in reality a complicated role. Sertoli cells form tight junctions with each other along their basal aspects that are apparently impermeable to blood cells and macromolecules. This structural arrangement constitutes the so-called blood-testis barrier. The contiguous layer of tight junctions defines basal and adluminal compartments. The spermatogonia occupy the basal compartment where they are exposed to blood levels of testosterone. The primary spermatocytes and subsequent stages of gametogenic cells occupy the adluminal compartment and are in intimate contact with or partially embedded within invaginations of the Sertoli cell plasma membrane. Important functions of the Sertoli cell includes nutritive support of the developing gametes, phagocytosis of residual bodies and degenerated gametes, protection of the genetically different spermatogenic cells from the immune system and secretion of various products including androgen-binding protein.

Sertoli cells are recognized by their basal location and their morphologic characteristics which includes the presence of a large pale nucleus enclosed by a convoluted nuclear envelope and a prominent nucleolus. Ultrastructurally, a well-developed Golgi apparatus, abundant SER, collections of thin microfilaments and peculiar inclusions (crystalloids) are seen.

The interstitium of the testis lies between the seminiferous tubules. Present are connective tissue cells and fibers; vascular, lymphatic and nervous elements; and a specific cell type, the Leydig cell. The Leydig cells are large and usually occur in small groups. By light microscopy, an abundant vacuolated cytoplasm is present. Peculiar rod-shaped crystalloid inclusions (of Reinke) may be observed in the cytoplasm along with lipofuscin granules. The former inclusions are of unknown functional significance, the latter increase in number with age. The nucleus (occasionally two) is characterized by the presence of a coarse chromatin pattern and usually a single distinct nucleolus. By EM, abundant SER and mitochondria with tubular cristae are present. Vacuoles observed by light microscopy prove ultrastructurally to be lipid droplets. Leydig cells produce testosterone under the influence of pituitary LH (ICSH).

## Excretory Ducts

The seminiferous tubules converge in the mediastinum where they eventually are lined by a single layer of modified Sertoli cells that are columnar in shape. Terminations of the seminiferous tubules open into the first (tubuli recti) of a series of excretory ducts that bear different names and structural characteristics.

1) Tubuli recti - in these straight tubules the lining epithelium becomes more cuboidal and the tubular diameter is decreased. Tubuli recti connect with the rete testis in the mediastinum.

2) Rete testis - consists of a labyrinthine network of anastomosing tubular channels. The height of the lining epithelium varies from squamous to columnar but typically is cuboidal and occasionally a cilium may be seen on the apical surface of some cells.

3) Ductuli efferentes - some 10-12 convoluted ductules that leave the rete to connect with the head of the epididymis. Lining cells may possess short apical microvilli (principal) cells or true cilia (ciliated cells). The height of the cells varies along the luminal surface resulting in a stellate configuration of the lumen in cross section. A thin layer of circularly arranged smooth muscle surrounds each ductule.

4) Ductus epididymidis (epididymis) - this is the first single duct. It runs a highly tortuous course and is continuous with the ductus deferens. A head, body and tail are recognized. The lining epithelium, unlike that of the efferent ductules, is uniform in height and consists of pseudostratified stratified columnar cells. Cells that reach the lumen display long microvillus processes (stereocilia). The muscular coat gradually increases in thickness and number of layers from the head to the tail to blend with that of the successive ductus deferens. The spermatozoa are stored here (mostly in the tail). As they are moved along the length of the duct, they gain functional capability. (Sperm from the head are nonmotile and incapable of fertilization whereas sperm from the head display both characteristics.) Other functions include resorption of the bulk of testicular fluid and the expulsion of sperm into the ductus deferens during ejaculation.

5) Ductus deferens (vas deferens) - of all tubular structures, the vas has perhaps the greatest relative wall thickness in comparison to luminal size. It consists of three layers: mucosa, muscularis and adventitia. The epithelium is similar to that of the terminal epididymis but is thrown up into longitudinal folds. Stereocilia are present particularly in the

proximal portions. The muscular coat is quite thick and consist of a thin inner longitudinal layer, a robust middle circular layer and an outer well-developed longitudinal layer. The function of the ductus deferens is to propel the sperm during ejaculation. The vas deferens terminates in an enlarged region, the ampulla. At the ampulla it is joined by the seminal vesicle to form an ejaculatory duct that passes through the prostate gland to enter the prostatic urethra at the colliculus seminalis (verumontanum).

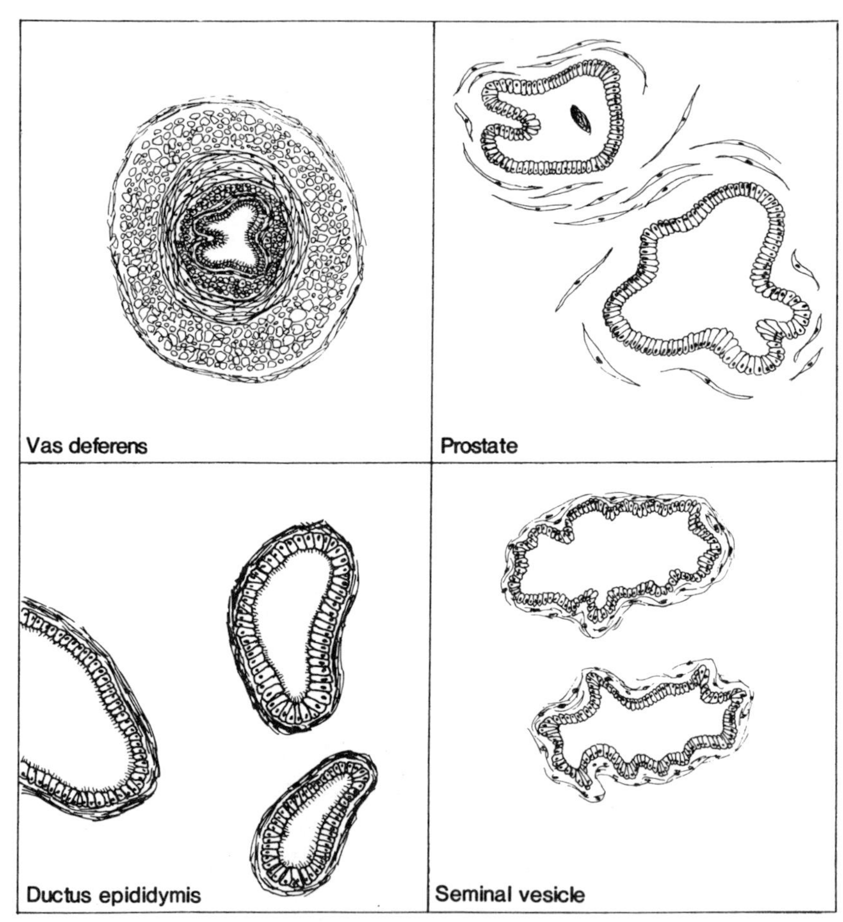


**Fig. 3.39.** Comparison of male ducts and accessory glands. (Courtesy Dr. R. Snell)

### Accessory Glands

The accessory glands include the seminal vesicles, prostate and bulbourethral glands.

## Seminal Vesicles

The seminal vesicle is a highly coiled tube. The wall consists of an external layer of connective tissue, a muscular coat of indistinct inner circular and outer longitudinal layers and a complex, highly folded mucosa. The epithelium lining the folds is pseudostratified columnar consisting of both secretory and basal cells. The secretory cells produce a viscous, yellowish secretion that contains fructose, ascorbate, citrate and prostaglandins. The seminal vesicle does not store sperm but adds nutritive and bioactive substances to the seminal fluid during ejaculation to enhance sperm viability and function.

## Prostate

The prostate completely surrounds the proximal portion of the urethra and is covered externally by a fibroelastic capsule. This contained portion of urethra is termed the prostatic urethra. Multiple ducts of some 30 to 50 compound tubuloalveolar glands that comprise the glandular component drain into the prostatic urethra.

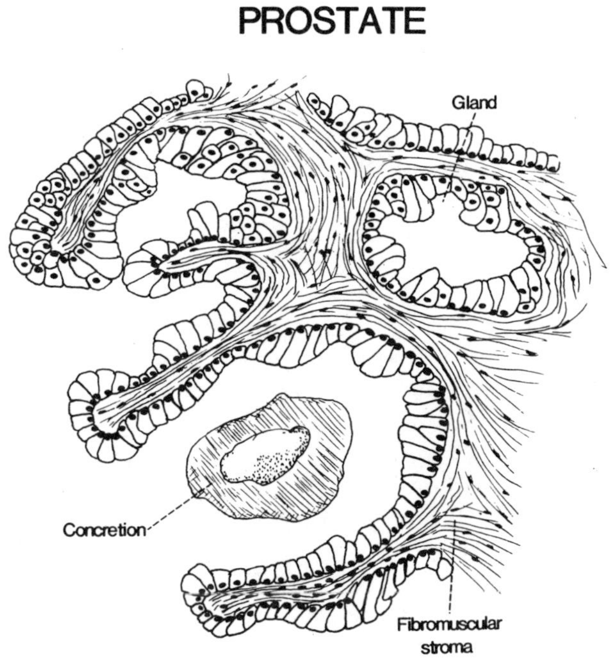

**PROSTATE**



**Fig. 3.40.** Structure of the prostate gland.

The glands are lined by a simple or pseudostratified columnar epithelium depending on glandular activity or the region within the organ. Secretory tubules and alveoli vary considerably in size and outline. Epithelial folding results in an irregular shape of the glandular lumina. Occasional intraglandular concretions (corpora amylacea) are present. Separating the glands is a characteristic fibromuscular stroma.

The glands produce a thin, slightly acidic and colorless secretion that contains abundant acid phosphatase activity, citrate, proteolytic enzymes and zinc. The proteolytic enzymes, especially fibrinolysin, may aid in liquefaction of semen.

## Bulbourethral Glands

Cowper's glands are small compound tubuloalveolar glands lined by a cuboidal to columnar epithelium. Both smooth muscle cells and skeletal muscle fibers occur within the stroma. The secretion is clear and viscous and has a high carbohydrate concentration. The secretions are thought to lubricate the urethrae prior to ejaculation.

## Penis

The penis consists of three cylindrical masses of erectile tissue bound together by a fibrous capsule, the tunica albuginea penis. The dorsal paired structures are termed the corpora cavernosa while the single ventral body containing the penile urethra is called the corpus spongiosum. The corpus spongiosum expands distally into the glands penis. The erectile tissue consists of a labyrinthine arrangement of thin endothelially lined channels (cavernous sinuses) supplied with blood by the helicine arteries.

Erotic stimulation results in loss of muscular tonus in the tunica media of the helicine arteries so that blood flows into the cavernous sinuses more rapidly than venous drainage can remove it. This process is potentiated by the compression of the relatively larger outer venous channels against the tunica albuginea reducing vascular outflow still further. The tunica albuginea is thinner around the corpus spongiosum and contains elastic fibers and a layer of circular smooth muscle. These structural modifications are important in assuring the patency of the penile urethra so that ejaculation is not compromised. When the evoking or subsequent stimuli are removed, the smooth muscle of the arteries regain tone and blood flow into the erectile bodies decreases. The slowly equilibrating venous drainage results in detumescence of the penis.

# FEMALE REPRODUCTIVE SYSTEM

The female reproductive system includes the ovaries, a series of interconnected tubular structures (fallopian tubes, uterus, vagina), the external genitalia and the breasts. The breasts were discussed previously in the integumentary system.

## Ovary

The ovary, like the testis, is a composite organ. It functions both as an exocrine and an endocrine gland. Its exocrine product is in the form of cells (oocytes) while its endocrine secretions are steroid hormones, largely estrogen, progesterone and related compounds.

The ovary is divided into an outer cortex and central medulla. It is surrounded externally by a layer of cuboidal cells, the germinal epithelium. At one time this layer was thought to be the production site of germ cells. It is now known to represent a structurally modified mesothelium. The germinal epithelium rests on a basement membrane and covers the outer connective tissue investment of the ovary, the tunica albuginea. The medulla contains a characteristic compact, highly cellular stroma which continues upward into the cortex to separate the chief cortical structures, the ovarian follicles.

### Follicular Development

At birth, nearly a million oocytes, each surrounded by a single layer of flattened cells to form a primordial follicle, are present. By puberty, only 40-50 thousand of these remain, the rest lost to normal attrition. With the onset of puberty and under the influence of pituitary gonadotrophins, the menstrual cycle is established. Gonadotropin release during a single cycle has effects on the ovary (follicular development and ovulation) which in turns affects the uterus (preparation for implantation). Implantation of a conceptus suspends the menstrual cycle and the gestational period commences. Cycling begins again following parturition. Lack of implantation results in menstruation.

During a human reproductive period, a single ovum is normally ovulated every 28 to 34 days by one of the ovaries. The selection of either the right or the left ovary seems to be a random event. In a typical reproductive period of about 36-40 years, only 400-500 ova are ovulated.

The cells that surround the ovum (follicular or granulosa cells) are influenced by gonadotropins to undergo a series of proliferative changes. Each month a number of follicles begin to develop but at slightly different rates. At any stage of maturation, a follicle may become atretic. Thus in the cortex of a reproductively competent female, follicles in various stages of development may be present with some of them continuing to mature

# FOLLICULAR DEVELOPMENT

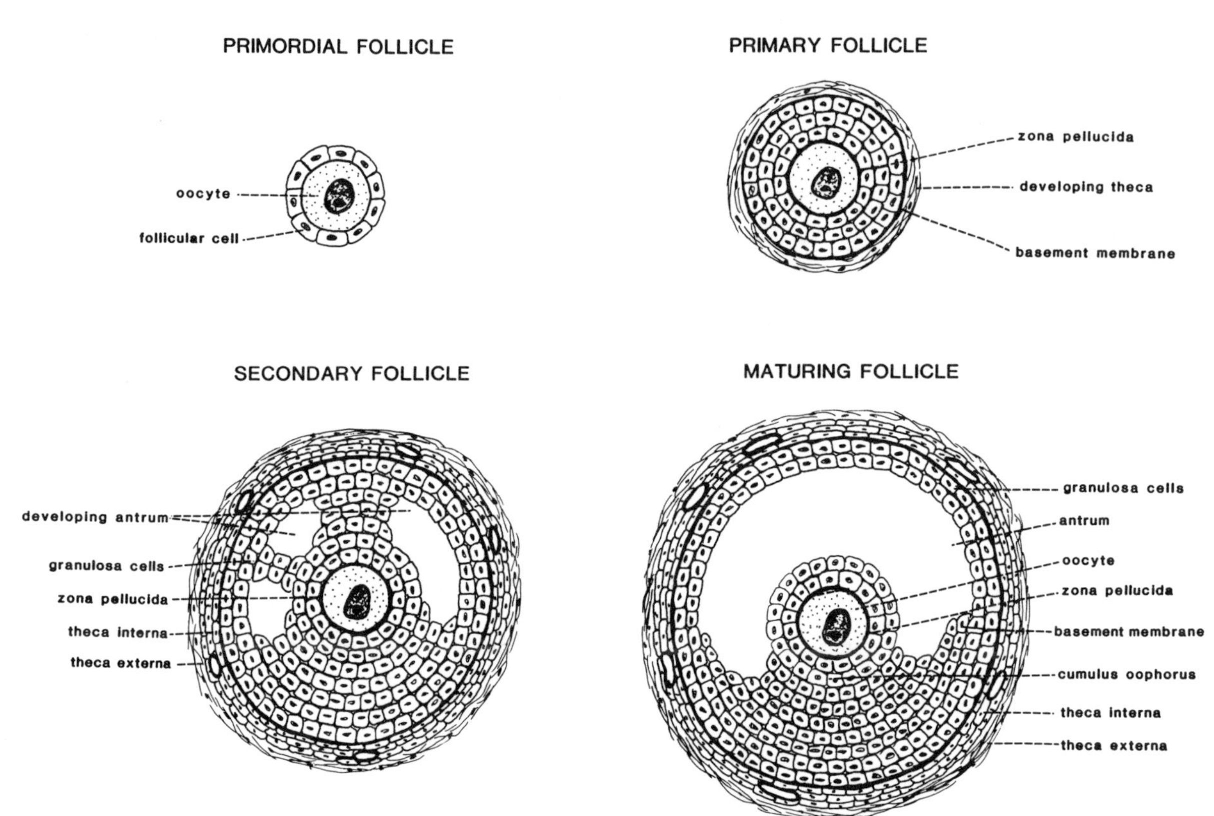


**Fig. 3.41.** Development of ovarian follicles.

while others are undergoing atresia. Normally only one follicle reaches functional maturity, the Graafian follicle. Others that have started to mature eventually degenerate. In the next menstrual cycle the process is repeated. It should be noted that follicular development occurs in both ovaries but that ovulation normally occurs in only one.

The developmental stages are recognized histologically as:

1) Primordial follicles - these are unilaminar follicles that are most numerous just below the tunica albuginea. They consist of an ovum surrounded by a single flattened layer of follicular cells. At this stage they seem to be refractory to the stimulating effects of gonadotropins.

2) Primary follicles - in these the oocyte is larger and the single layer of follicular cells is cuboidal and then divides to become a stratified layer of granulosa

cells. Between the ovum and the first layer of granulosa cells, a prominent layer of glycoprotein, the zona pellucida appears. A developing outer layer of ovarian stroma, the theca, begins to form. The later stages of primary follicles are sometimes termed preantral follicles.

3) Secondary (antral) follicles - when 6 or more layers of granulosa cells are present, the cells begin to produce a serous fluid that separates the cells. At first the separation results in only small spaces but these eventually coalesce into a single crescentic antral cavity or antrum. It is filled with a fluid, the liquor folliculi, that is somewhat viscous and contains hyaluronic acid. The ovum bulges into the antrum surrounded by a mass of granulosa cells, the cumulus oophorus. Cells directly in contact with the zona pellucida form a layer known as the corona radiata. Cell processes of the corona radiata pass through the zona pellucida to contact the surface of the ovary and possibly play a nutritive supporting role. Microvillus processes of the ovary pass into the zona pellucida. Granulosa cells not comprising the corona radiata or cumulus oophorus are collectively termed the membrana granulosa. Outside the basement membrane of the granulosa cells, the theca is composed of two layers, a vascular estrogen-producing theca interna and a fibrous theca externa.

4) Mature (Graafian) follicle - a single fully mature follicle occurs per menstrual cycle. Fluid begins to accumulate between the cells of the cumulus oophorus so that just before ovulation the ovum is freed into the fluid filled antrum surrounded only by the remaining corona radiata. The Graafian follicle is large, fills the entire thickness of the cortex, and bulges from the surface of the ovary.

## Ovulation

A surge in the release of LH by the pituitary at midcycle results in the subsequent (24 to 36 hours later) rupture of the follicle. At rupture, the ovum is transferred into the fallopian tube. The ovum which has been suspended in the first meiotic dictyotene stage of prophase since it was first established in the ovary during fetal life now completes the first meiotic division and proceeds to metaphase of the second meiotic division. Completion of the second meiotic division depends on the occurrence of fertilization. The ovum is capable of being fertilized for about 24 hours. Fertilization usually occurs in the upper third of the fallopian tube with ascent into the uterus requiring 3 to 5 days. Implantation occurs only in a receptive (functionally differentiated) uterine endometrium.

## Corpus Luteum

At ovulation, the Graafian follicle collapses and some hemorrhage may occur. The remaining structure begins to function in an important endocrine role and is termed the corpus luteum. The basement membrane of the granulosa cells is lost and the layer of cells is vascularized. They begin to produce steroids (progesterone) and are termed the granulosa lutein cells. The theca interna cells continue to secrete estrogen and are now called the theca lutein cells.

If conception and implantation occur, the corpus luteum will continue to function as the corpus luteum of pregnancy. If fertilization fails, function of the corpus luteum continues some 10 to 12 days followed by degeneration ultimately into a large eosinophilic body known as a corpus albicans.

## Fallopian Tube

The fallopian (uterine) tube is a long muscular tube composed of four parts: the funnel-shaped fimbriated infundibulum; a long intermediate segment, the ampulla; a narrow segment just outside the uterine wall termed the isthmus and an intramural segment, the pars uterina or pars interstitialis. The histology of these segments varies somewhat but in common the wall is composed of three layers. The mucosa is thrown up into a

FALLOPIAN TUBE

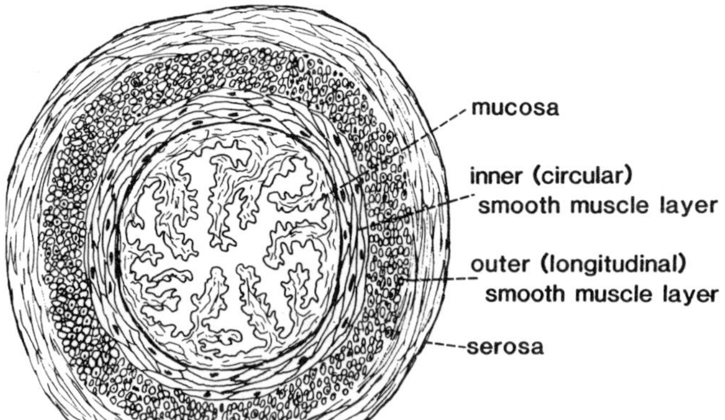

mucosa
inner (circular) smooth muscle layer
outer (longitudinal) smooth muscle layer
serosa

**Fig. 3.42.** Fallopian tube structure. (Courtesy Dr. R. Snell)

labyrinthine complex of longitudinal folds. The folds are branched and supported by a core of vascularized connective tissue. The epithelium is simple, low-columnar. Cilia may be present on the apical surface. It is said that some cilia beat toward the ovary while others beat in the direction of the uterus. This arrangement may be useful in movement of the sperm and ovum respectively. The relatively thick muscularis comprises an inner circular and outer longitudinal layer of smooth muscle. The uterine tube is covered externally by a serosa.

## Uterus

The uterus is composed of a body (fundus) from which projects a narrow structure, the cervix. The uterine lumen continues through the cervix as the endocervical canal. The cervix is continuous with the vagina. Three coats comprise the uterus.

1) Perimetrium - the uterus proper is covered externally by a serosa.

2) Myometrium - is the thickest layer and is composed of a feltwork pattern of smooth muscle. During pregnancy both hypertrophy and hyperplasia of the smooth muscle cells occur.

3) Endometrium - is lined by a simple columnar epithelium over a lamina propria. Many simple or occasionally branched tubular glands extend from the surface to the level of the underlying myometrium. Two functionally distinct layers occur. The layer just above the myometrium is termed the stratum basalis, is not affected by cyclic changes and persists during menstruation and parturition. It is considered a reserve layer. Above is a layer termed the stratum functionalis. It is affected by the cycle changes that occur with the menstrual cycle and is lost with menstruation and parturition. It may be subdivided into a superficial stratum compactum and an underlying stratum spongiosa.

### Cyclic Changes of the Endometrium

During the reproductive period, the uterus undergoes a series of changes that are correlated with the maturation of the ovarian follicles, ovulation and the function of the corpus luteum. Proliferative and secretory changes occur under hormonal control in preparation for implantation. If implantation fails, then regressive changes occur as a result of ischemia.

1) Menstrual phase - coiled arteries in the stratum functionalis constrict rendering the outer layers of the endometrium ischemic. Loss of the outer endometrial glands, blood and uterine fluid into the vagina

occurs. The stratum basalis is retained because it is supplied by straight or basal arteries that are not dependent on hormonal support. (Vida infra).

2) Proliferative phase - mitotic activity in the stratum basalis begins to reconstitute the endometrial lining so that eventually a series of long straight parallel glands are formed. This phase is dependent on estrogen produced by the developing follicles.

3) Secretory phase - following ovulation and under hormonal influence of the developing corpus luteum, the glands increase significantly in thickness and assume a corkscrew configuration. The glands begin to secrete small amounts of a glycogen rich product and mucous. It is during this phase that implantation may occur.

4) Premenstrual phase - if fertilization fails, the corpus luteum degenerates and with loss of progesterone support the coiled arteries in the stratum functionalis begin periodic constriction. The functionalis decreases in thickness largely as a result of water loss. Once the ischemia is severe and prolonged enough to cause degeneration and sloughing, the menstrual phase begins.

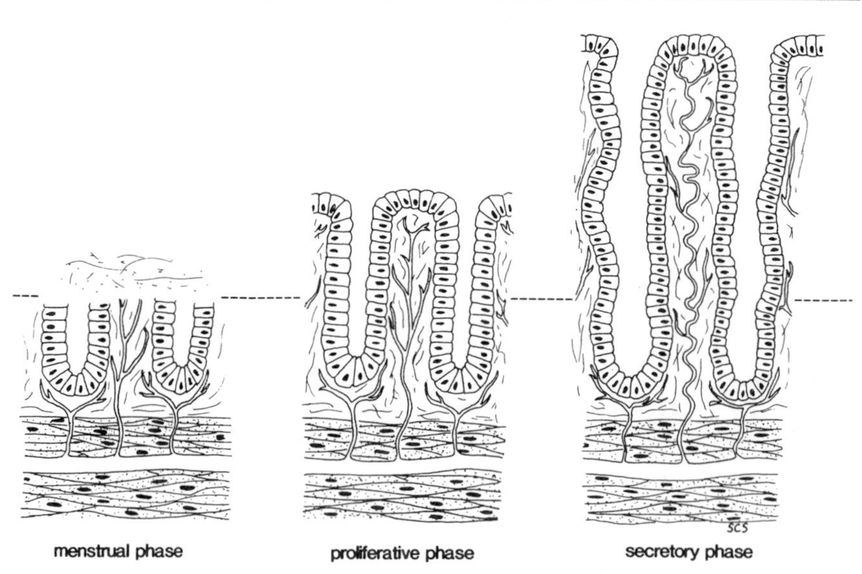


**Fig. 3.43.** Uterine mucosa in different phases of the menstrual cycle. (Courtesy Dr. R. Snell)

## Cervix

The cervix contains a central lumen, the cervical canal or endocervix, which communicates with the uterine cavity at the internal os and with the vagina at the external os. The cervix is composed mostly of dense connective tissue with smaller amounts of smooth muscle. The outer face of the cervix is a transitional zone from the mucous secreting simple columnar epithelium of the endocervix to the moist stratified squamous epithelium of the vagina.

## Vagina

There are no glands in the vagina. The surface epithelium is of the moist stratified squamous variety rich in glycogen. The vaginal epithelium is influenced by estrogen (cornification) during the menstrual cycle. Beneath the mucosa is a predominately longitudinal arrangement of smooth muscle to form a thin, indistinct muscularis. The outer layer is termed the fibrosa and consists of fairly dense fibrous connective tissue.

## SPECIAL SENSE ORGANS

### Vision - the Eye

The major layers of the eye include the corneoscleral coat (tunica fibrosa), the uvea (tunica vasculosa) and the retina (tunica interna).

#### Corneoscleral Coat

1) Sclera - is a tough, thick (0.5 mm) coat continuous anteriorly with the cornea. The tendons of the extraocular muscles insert on the sclera.

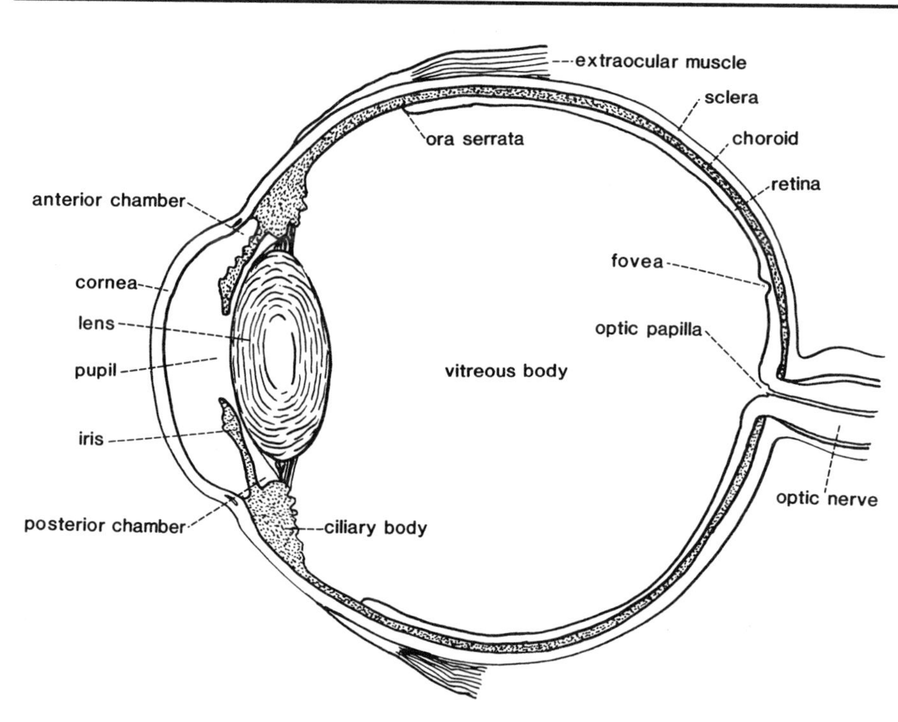


**Fig. 3.44.** Structure of the eye.

2) Cornea - a transparent, avascular layer which consists of 5 layers. From the inside to the outside these are:

   a) Nonkeratinizing stratified squamous <u>epithelium</u> approximately 5 to 7 layers thick. It has very good healing capacity.
   b) <u>Bowman's membrane</u> consists of basement membrane material of the layer above and a thin layer of densely packed collagen fibers.

c) Substantia propria or stroma is the major component of the cornea and consists of parallel collagen fibrils and ground substance of chondroitin sulfate and keratan sulfate. It is avascular.

d) Descemet's membrane is a thin (10 micron), acellular layer of elastin and basement membrane material from the layer below.

e) Endothelium is a single layer of cuboidal cells.

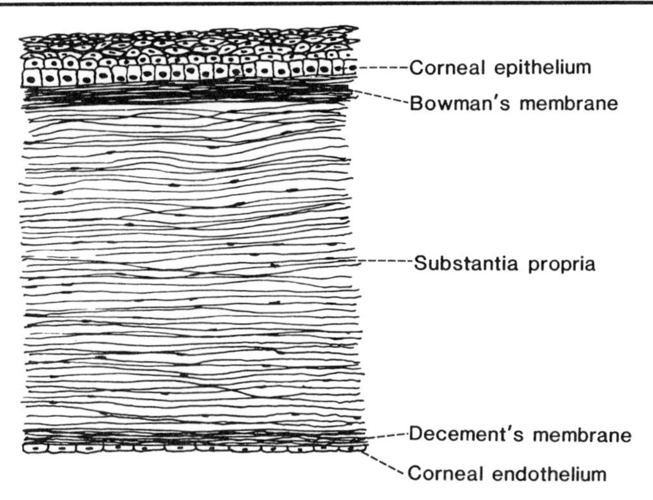


**Fig. 3.45.** Layers of the cornea.

3) Limbus - is the zone of transition between cornea and sclera.

## Uvea

1) Choroid - a pigmented layer of epithelial cells resting on a basement membrane (Bruch's membrane) and an underlying heavily pigmented and vascularized connective tissue.

2) Ciliary body - extends from ora serrata to beginning of iris. Contains pigmented epithelium, vascularized connective tissue and smooth muscle cells, the ciliary muscle, which adjusts the shape of the lens.

3) Iris - contains the pupil and adjusts its size. A circularly oriented sphincter muscle and a radially arranged dilatory muscle are found here. The cells of these muscles are modified epithelial cells that are capable of contraction (myoepithelial cells). Pigment present in the iris results in eye coloration.

Retina

1) Pigmented epithelium.
2) Outer segments of rods and cones.
3) External limiting membrane.
4) Outer nuclear layer.
5) Outer plexiform layer.
6) Inner nuclear layer.
7) Inner plexiform layer.
8) Ganglion cell layer.
9) Optic nerve fiber layer.
10) Internal limiting membrane.

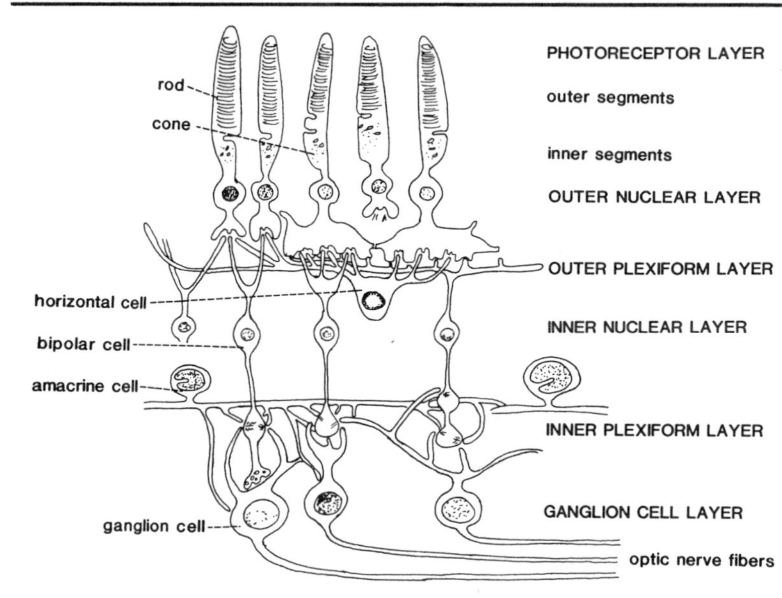


**Fig. 3.46.** Layers of the retina.

The photoreceptor cells of the eye are the rods and cones. Each rod or cone consists of an outer segment which is connected to the inner segment by a narrow stalk. The outer segment contains a stack of membranous disks. Outer segments of rods are cylindrical in shape while the cone outer segments are conical. Outer segments are highly modified cilia and the rod and cone cells are modified neural cells that convert photic energy into a generator potential which depolarizes contacting nerve cell fibers of the optic nerve. This conversion occurs via photosensitive pigments that are located in the membranous disks of the outer segments. The pigment of rods is known as rhodopsin while that of cones is called iodopsin. These pigments are produced in the inner segments in an area known as the ellipsoid. The base of the cone is known as the pedicle while the corresponding region of the rod is known as the spherule.

The cells of Muller are supporting cells (glia) of the

retina that extend from the rods and cones at the external limiting membrane to the internal limiting membrane. Their nuclei are located in the inner nuclear layer.

RETINAL PHOTORECEPTOR CELLS

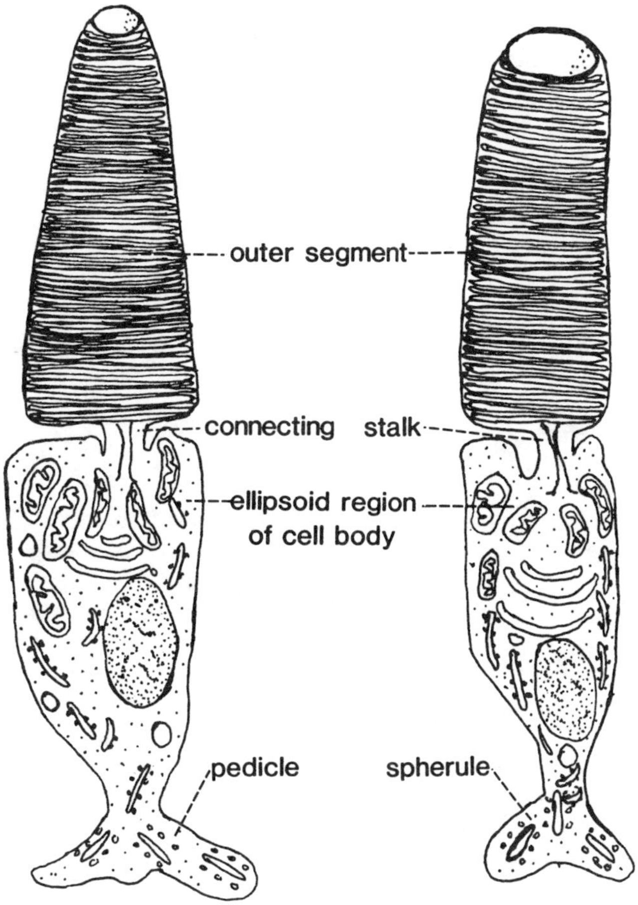

outer segment
connecting stalk
ellipsoid region of cell body
pedicle
spherule
CONE
ROD

**Fig. 3.47.** Comparison of a rod and cone.

### Hearing and Balance - The Ear

Hearing is dependent upon the funneling action of the external ear, the tympanic membrane and the proper function of the three ossicles of the middle ear. The sensory neuroepithelial cells for both hearing and balance are located in the inner ear. Some of these are present in the sensory organ of hearing (organ of Corti) whereas others that respond to changes in the position of the head or to linear or rotational motion are located in the membranous labyrinth.

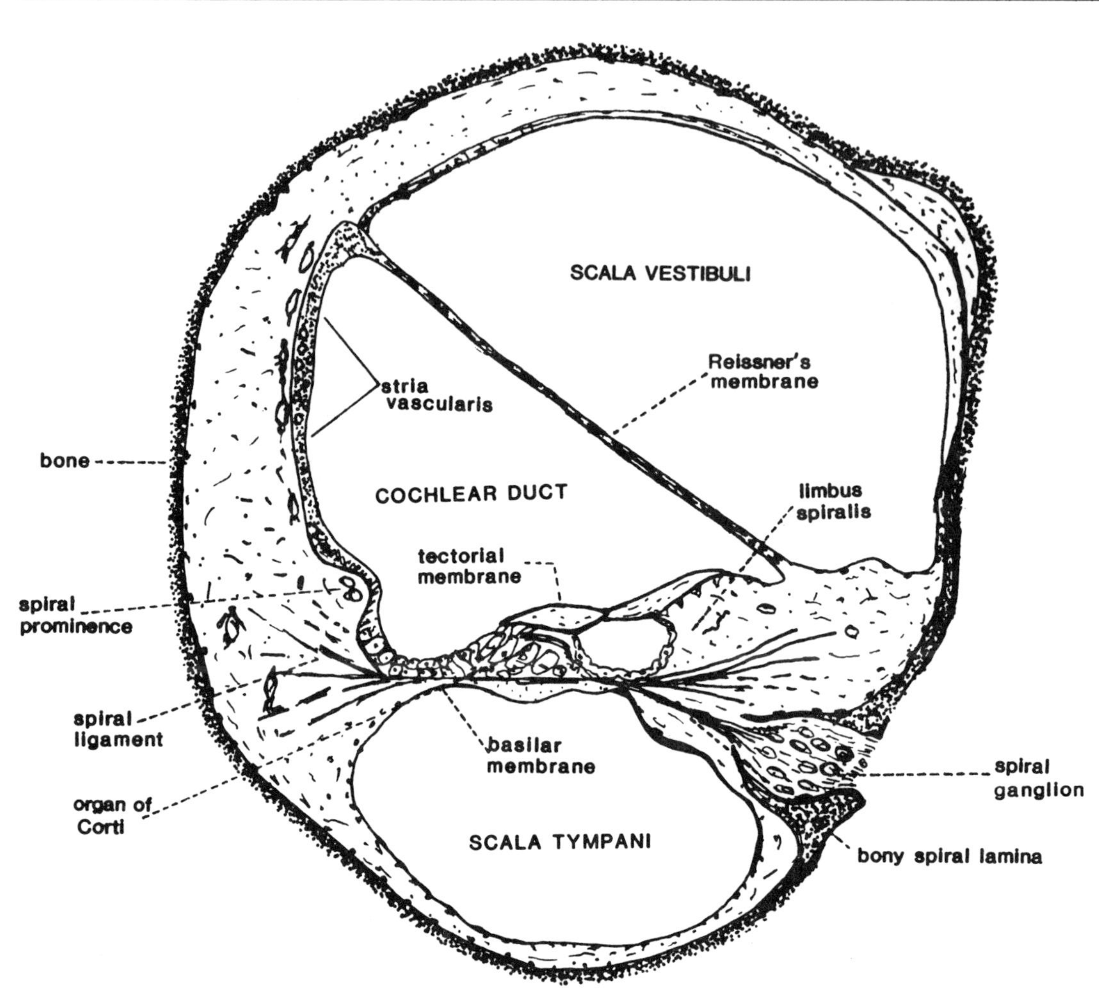


**Fig. 3.48.** The cochlea.

## Cochlear Duct

Also termed the scala media, it is contained within the bony cochlea. This duct is represented by a canal that spirals some two and a half times around the central modiolus. The cochlear duct is filled with a fluid known as endolymph. This fluid is compositionally different that the fluid (perilymph) filling the chambers above and below, the scala vestibuli and scala tympani. Within the cochlear duct is the organ of hearing, the organ of Corti.

## Organ of Corti

This structure contains important epithelial transducers, the hair cells. These cells are capable of transforming mechanical vibrations of the basilar membrane into nervous impulses which are relayed via the cochlear nerve to the bipolar nerve cell bodies in the spiral ganglion within the bony modiolus.

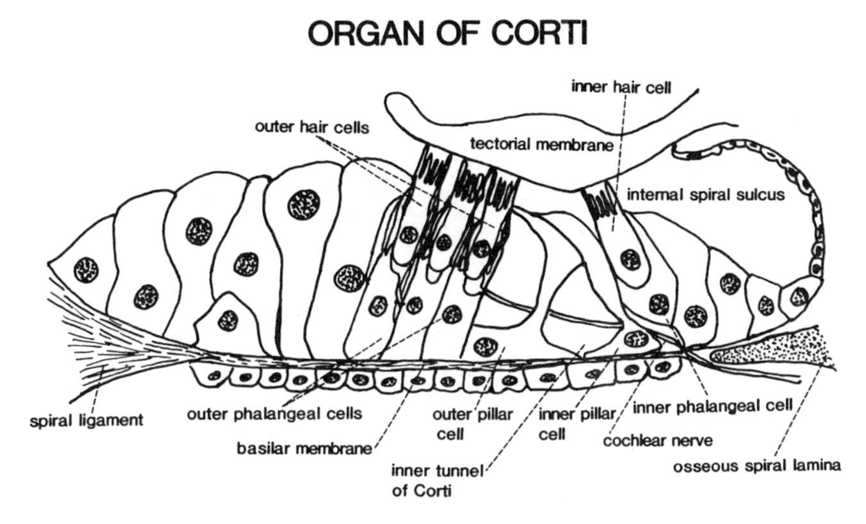


**Fig. 3.49.** Organ of Corti.

## Membranous Labyrinth

The three semicircular canals, the anterior saccule and the posterior utricle are filled with endolymph and are separated by the surrounding closely apposed bone (osseous labyrinth) by a layer of perilymph.

An expanded portion of each semicircular canal, the ampulla, contains a crista or group of neuroepithelial (hair) cells. A gelatinous mass, the cupula, overlies each crista. Changes in angular acceleration of the head alters the position of the cupula and results in stimulation of the hair cells and the generation of a nervous impulse which is relayed by way of the vestibular nerve.

The utricle and saccule also contain neuroepithelial cells in the form of a macula. Hair cells of the macula are covered superiorly by a gelatinous material (otolithic membrane) containing calcium carbonate-protein crystals (otoconia). Alteration of the position of the otolithic membrane occurring with positional changes in the head with respect to gravity stimulates the hair cells to generate an action potential in connecting nerve fibers.

## Smell - The Olfactory Mucosa

The olfactory mucosa consists of a pseudostratified columnar epithelium slightly thicker than the respiratory epithelium of the nasal cavity. The olfactory receptor cells are modified bipolar neurons. They are surrounded and supported by sustentacular cells. The latter bear apically placed nuclei and surface microvilli. Short basal cells (reserve cells) rest on the basement membrane but fail to reach the apical surface. The olfactory cells contain a modified apical dendrite which ends in a bulb-like structure, the olfactory knob. From the olfactory knob, originate several nonmotile cilia which are the olfactory receptor organelles. The axons of olfactory cells extend through the basement membrane to join those of many others and to eventually enter the olfactory bulbs via the cribriform plate of the ethmoid bone. In olfactory reception there is no epithelial transducer cell, the modified bipolar neuron or olfactory cell is chemically stimulated to generate a nervous impulse.

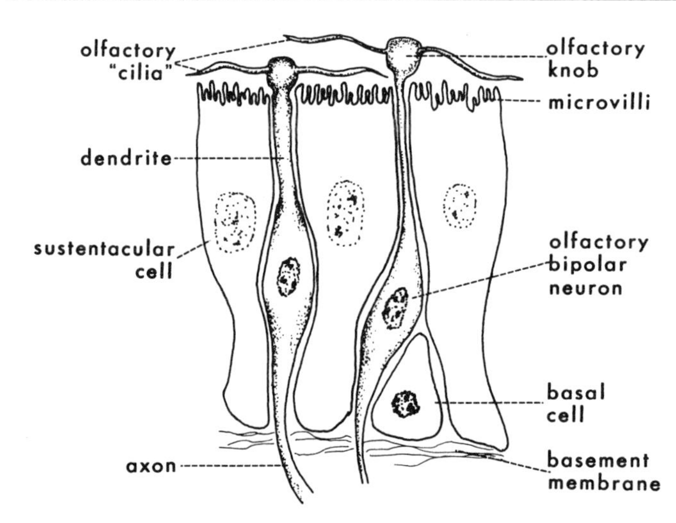


**Fig. 3.50.** Olfactory mucosa.

## Taste - Taste Buds

The organ of taste is rather diffuse and is represented by the taste buds found in association with the fungiform and circumvallate papillae of the tongue and outside the tongue within the soft palate, epiglottis and posterior pharyngeal wall. Taste buds are microscopic structures which rest on the epithelial (moist stratified squamous) basement membrane and extend to the free surface. They are composed of two major cells types which are arranged alternately with each other like the staves of a barrel. The neuroepithelial (sensory) cells are light-staining when compared with the hyperchromatic sustentacular cells. Both types of cells possess apical microvilli (hairs) which circumscribe the apical pore. Nerve fibers are found in association with the neuroepithelial cells of the taste buds. Chemical stimulation of taste buds results in the production of a generator potential which results in induction of a nervous impulse in the associated nerve fibers.

## TASTE BUD

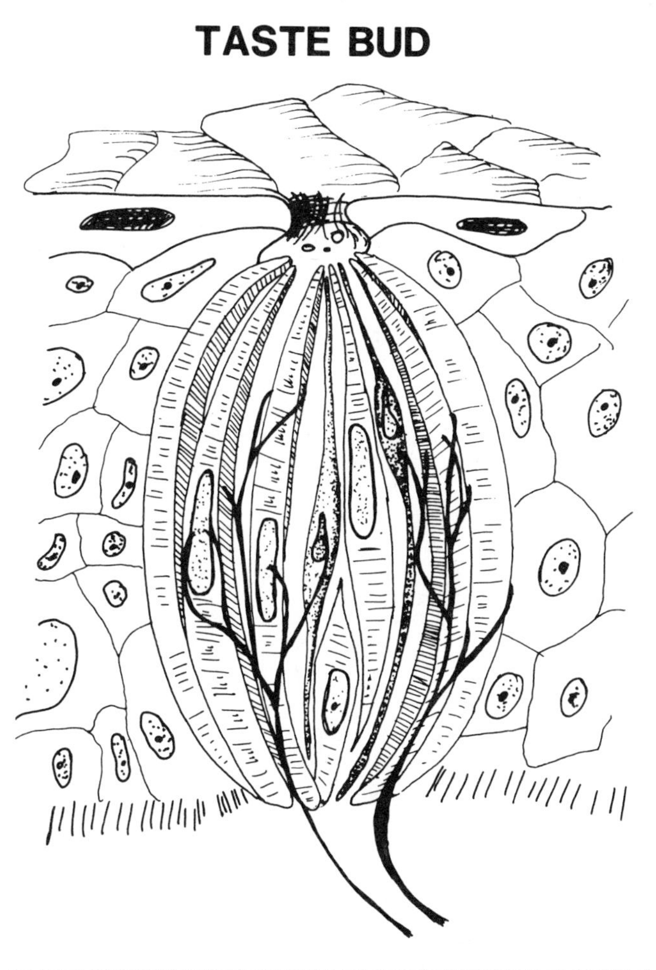

Fig. 3.51. A taste bud.

### Touch -Cutaneous Sensory Receptors

Touch is not considered a special sense. It afferent input to the CNS is via general somatic afferent (GSA) fibers. Free nerve endings (not associated with other cells) are particularly prominent in the skin but are also present in the mucous membranes and cornea. Different fibers are capable of receiving sensations of light touch, pain and thermal changes. The free nerve endings associated with hairs (peritrichial endings) are particularly sensitive receptors.

Other nerve endings are associated with specialized epithelial cells such as the Merkel cell in the epidermis. In this association, so-called Merkel discs are formed which are believed to be a type of mechanoreceptor. Some Merkel discs are capable of responding to vibratory stimuli.

A third category of cutaneous sensory receptors are known as encapsulated nerve endings. These include:

1) Pacinian corpuscles - are large, lamellated bodies. They are particularly prominent in the subcutaneous tissue of the fingertips, palms and soles but may be found in many other locations throughout the body. They contain a single nerve fiber and respond to pressure and vibration.

2) Meissner's corpuscles - are found in the dermal papillae of the digits, lips, nipples and external genitalia. Two or more nerve fibers enter these structures which respond to touch and allow two-point tactile discrimination.

3) Ruffini's corpuscles and Krause's end bulbs - are located in the subcutis and respond to mechanical deformation.

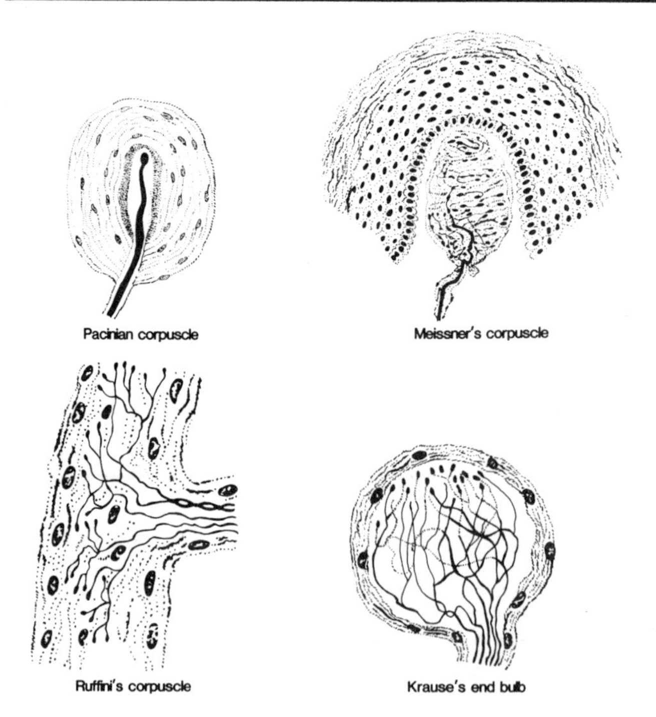


**Fig. 3.52.** Encapsulated sensory endings.

## UNIT III: PROFICIENCY EXAM

**DIRECTIONS:** For the following questions select the one best answer which completes the statement or answers the question.

1) Synaptic connections between neurons are common in all of the following areas EXCEPT:
   A. Sensory ganglia.
   B. Autonomic ganglia.
   C. Cerebral cortex.
   D. Cerebellar cortex.
   E. Gray matter of the spinal cord.

2) Myelin:
   A. Is absent in most large peripheral nerves.
   B. Of the central nervous system is formed by Schwann cells.
   C. Is composed of concentric layers of plasma membrane wrapped "jelly roll" around the axon.
   D. Normally covers the perikaryon as well as the processes (axons and dendrites).
   E. All of the above.

3) The adventitial layer of large arteries may contain:
   A. Nerve trunks.
   B. Arterioles.
   C. Autonomic ganglia.
   D. Lymphatic vessels.
   E. All of the above.

4) The so-called "striations" of striated ducts in salivary glands are related to the presence of:
   A. A basally located Golgi complex.
   B. Numerous attachment plaques and associated tonofibrils.
   C. Parallel arrangement of the cisternae of the endoplasmic reticulum.
   D. A combination of radially arranged mitochondria and basal infoldings of the plasma membrane.
   E. Multiple, regularly arranged and prominent microvilli.

5) The appendix:
   A. Is similar to the duodenum in histologic appearance.
   B. Lacks lymph nodules.
   C. Contains argentaffin cells.
   D. Lacks goblet cells.
   E. Secretes HCl.

6) The ameloblast is the cell that:
   A. Maintains dentin.
   B. Forms dentin.
   C. Maintains enamel.
   D. Forms enamel.
   E. Lines the dental pulp.

7) The synthesis of glucocorticoids (cortisol) is associated with the:
   A. Zona glomerulosa.
   B. Zona fasciculata.
   C. Zona reticularis.
   D. Zona fasciculata and zona reticularis.
   E. Medullary cells.

8) As the ovarian follicle grows and matures, the oocyte becomes located in a mound of follicular cells called the:
   A. Call-Exner body.
   B. Cumulus oophorus.
   C. Stratum compactum.
   D. Zona pellucida.
   E. Antral cavity.

9) The cells of the testis which are <u>directly</u> affected by or acted upon by FSH are the:
   A. Leydig cells.
   B. Spermatogonia.
   C. Primary spermatocytes.
   D. Sertoli cells.
   E. Myoid cells.

10) Since the liver is metabolically very active, which cytoplasmic organelle would be expected in large numbers?
   A. Golgi apparatus.
   B. Lysosomes.
   C. Rough endoplasmic reticulum.
   D. Mitochondria.
   E. Microbodies.

11) Cell bodies of sensory neurons located in the olfactory mucosa are:
   A. Unipolar.
   B. Bipolar.
   C. Multipolar.
   D. Anaxonic.
   E. None of the above.

12) Intracellular canaliculi are best represented in the:
- A. Keratinocytes of the epidermis.
- B. Kupffer cells in the liver.
- C. Oxyphil cells in the parathyroid.
- D. Gastric parietal cells.
- E. Gastric chief cells.

13) Tonsils are characterized by the:
- A. Presence of a well-developed connective tissue capsule over the entire surface.
- B. Close physical relationship to epithelial surfaces.
- C. Presence of afferent lymphatic vessels.
- D. Presence of Billroth's cords.
- E. Absence of germinal centers.

14) The cell bodies of spinal, cranial and autonomic ganglia are surrounded or encapsulated by:
- A. Oligodendroglia cells.
- B. Ependymal cells.
- C. Satellite cells.
- D. Astrocytes.
- E. Microglial cells.

15) The first portion of the conducting division of the respiratory tract to lack mural cartilage is the:
- A. Trachea.
- B. Primary bronchus.
- C. Segmental bronchus.
- D. Bronchiole.
- E. Alveolar duct.

16) The great alveolar cells (type II pneumocytes):
- A. Are also known as pulmonary alveolar macrophages.
- B. Secrete surfactant.
- C. Are chemoreceptor cells (sensitive to $O_2$ levels of inspired air).
- D. Are baroreceptor cells (sensitive to pulmonary blood pressure levels).
- E. None of the above.

17) The parafollicular cells (C-cells) of the thyroid gland:
- A. Possess an iodine pump in their plasma membrane.
- B. Secrete thyroglobulin into the thyroid follicles.
- C. Remove thyroglobulin from the thyroid follicles .
- D. Secrete tri- and tetraiodothyronine into adjacent perivascular structures.
- E. None of the above.

18) The most common cell type in the islets of Langerhans is the:
A. A-cell.
B. B-cell.
C. C-cell.
D. D-cell.
E. Centroacinar cell.

19) The endometrial layer(s) lost during menstruation and parturition are the:
A. Stratum basalis only.
B. Stratum spongiosum only.
C. Stratum compactum.
D. Stratum compactum and stratum spongiosum.
E. Stratum spongiosum and stratum basalis.

20) Morphologically, the vagina is characterized by:
A. A well-developed muscularis mucosae.
B. Exhibiting many mucous secreting glands in the lamina propria.
C. A lining of moist stratified squamous epithelium.
D. A lining of simple columnar epithelium with goblet cells but lacking absorptive cells.
E. None of the above.

21) Pepsinogen does not become a functional enzyme until exposed to the secretions of the:
A. Parietal cell.
B. Chief cell.
C. Mucous neck cell.
D. Paneth cell.
E. None of the above.

22) The kidney plays a role in:
A. Maintaining blood volume.
B. Adjusting blood pH.
C. Removal of waste metabolites.
D. Adjusting blood osmolarity.
E. All of the above.

23) The hormone renin is produced by the:
A. Juxtaglomerular cells.
B. Cells of the macula densa.
C. Mesangial cells.
D. Glomerular endothelial cells.
E. Podocytes.

24) The visceral layer of Bowman's capsule is formed by:
A. Kupffer cells.
B. Capillary endothelium.
C. Transitional epithelium.
D. Podocytes.
E. Cap cells.

25) The capillaries in the cerebral cortex are:
A. Sinusoidal.
B. Continuous without fenestrations.
C. Continuous with fenestra covered by diaphragms.
D. Continuous with uncovered fenestra.
E. None of the above.

26) Pituitary basophils are believed to produce all of the following hormones EXCEPT:
A. Follicle stimulating hormone.
B. Luteinizing hormone.
C. Prolactin.
D. Adrenocorticotrophic hormone.
E. Melanocyte stimulating hormone.

27) The principle storage site for spermatozoa is thought to be the:
A. Epididymal duct.
B. Efferent ductules.
C. Proximal segment of the vas deferens.
D. Seminal vesicle.
E. Prostatic utricle.

28) The cells in the testis that provide nutritive support for the developing sperm are the:
A. Sertoli cells.
B. Seminiferous cells.
C. Gonadotrophs.
D. Leydig cells.
E. None of the above.

29) The layer of the heart that is homologous to the tunica intima is the:
A. Parietal pericardium.
B. Epicardium.
C. Myocardium.
D. Endocardium.
E. None of the above.

30) Veins which demonstrate longitudinal bundles of smooth muscle in their adventitia include:
A. Vena cava.
B. Portal vein.
C. Both.
D. Neither.

31) The parenchyma of an organ may consist of:
- A. General surfacing epithelium.
- B. Secretory or glandular epithelium.
- C. Nervous tissue.
- D. Skeletal muscle.
- E. Any of the above.

32) The valves of the heart are:
- A. Attached to the cardiac skeleton at the annuli fibrosi.
- B. Folds or duplications of the epicardium.
- C. Normally well-vascularized.
- D. Covered by mesothelium.
- E. All of the above.

33) The scala media (cochlear duct) is filled with:
- A. Air.
- B. Blood.
- C. Perilymph.
- D. Endolymph.
- E. None of the above.

34) The layer immediately beneath the corneal epithelium is:
- A. Bowman's membrane.
- B. Bowman's capsule.
- C. Substantia propria.
- D. Endothelium.
- E. Descemet's membrane.

35) Pacinian corpuscles:
- A. Contain a single nerve fiber.
- B. Are multilamellated.
- C. Are the largest encapsulated sensory receptors.
- D. Are stimulated by pressure.
- E. All of the above.

**CHANGE IN FORMAT:** For the following questions select:

- (A) if only 1, 2 and 3 are correct.
- (B) if only 1 and 3 are correct.
- (C) if only 2 and 4 are correct.
- (D) if only 4 is correct.
- (E) if all are correct.

36) Compact layers of circularly arranged smooth muscle is a characteristic feature of:
1. Medium sized veins.
2. Muscular arteries.
3. Venules.
4. Arterioles.

**(A) = 1, 2, 3 (B) = 1, 3 (C) = 2, 4 (D) = 4 only (E) = All**

37) Both the cerebral and cerebellar cortices:
1. Are comprised of neurons and glial cells.
2. Contain molecular, granular and ganglionic layers.
3. Consist of superficial layers of gray matter with underlying nerve cells processes forming white matter.
4. Contain very few multipolar neurons.

38) The white pulp of the spleen may contain:
1. Both B- and T- lymphocytes.
2. Small muscular arteries or arterioles.
3. Germinal centers.
4. Abundant lymph sinuses.

39) The type I pneumocyte:
1. Contains cytosomes which are visualized at the ultrastructural level as multilaminar bodies.
2. Produces a secretory product that is rich in phospholipid.
3. Produces a surface active material (surfactant).
4. Has an attenuated cytoplasm through which gaseous exchange occurs.

40) The secretion produced by the seminal vesicle is:
1. Viscous in nature.
2. Slightly alkaline.
3. Rich in fructose.
4. Rich in acid phosphatase.

41) Which of the following structures are part of the respiratory division of the lung?
1. Alveoli.
2. Alveolar ducts.
3. Respiratory bronchioles.
4. Terminal bronchioles.

42) The elastic component of elastic arteries is:
1. In the form of elastic fibers.
2. In the form of fenestrated elastic laminae.
3. Confined to the tunica intima.
4. Best represented in the tunica media.

43) Podocytes are found in the:
1. Macula densa.
2. Proximal convoluted tubule.
3. Juxtaglomerular apparatus.
4. Visceral layer of Bowman's capsule.

(A) = 1, 2, 3   (B) = 1, 3   (C) = 2, 4   (D) = 4 only   (E) = All

44) The parathyroid gland:
1. Of infants contains only one parenchymal cell type.
2. Responds to low blood levels of calcium by release of parathormone.
3. Of adults contains two types of parenchymal cells.
4. Is progressively infiltrated with fat with advancing age.

45) Which of the following are not encapsulated nerve endings?
1. Pacinian corpuscles.
2. Meissner's corpuscles.
3. Ruffini's corpuscles.
4. Merkel disks.

46) Which of the following structures would NOT be expected to contain striated ducts?
1. Sublingual glands.
2. Submandibular gland.
3. Parotid glands.
4. Pancreas (exocrine).

47) Afferent lymphatic vessels are associated with:
1. Palatine tonsil.
2. Lymph nodules.
3. Spleen.
4. Lymph nodes.

48) The endocardium is:
1. Thicker in the atrium than in the ventricle.
2. Thicker in the ventricle than in the atria.
3. Duplicated to form the valves.
4. Interrupted or discontinuous over the heart valves.

49) Components of the renal corpuscle that function as part of the filtration mechanism include:
1. Fenestrated capillaries.
2. Basal lamina.
3. Slit membrane.
4. Pedicles (foot processes) of podocytes.

50) Taste buds are found in association with the:
1. Fungiform papillae.
2. Circumvallate papillae.
3. Epiglottis.
4. Ventral surface of the tongue.

# EXAMS KEY

## PROFICIENCY EXAM: UNIT I

1. D
2. C
3. A
4. D
5. A
6. E
7. D
8. B
9. E
10. C
11. E
12. D
13. E
14. D
15. A
16. A
17. C
18. A
19. B
20. A
21. D
22. E
23. C
24. B
25. E

## PROFICIENCY EXAM: UNIT II

1. A
2. E
3. E
4. B
5. C
6. E
7. D
8. B
9. B
10. D
11. D
12. B
13. E
14. A
15. E
16. D
17. D
18. B
19. B
20. E
21. E
22. D
23. D
24. E
25. E
26. A
27. B
28. E
29. D
30. B
31. D
32. C
33. B
34. A
35. D
36. A
37. A
38. C
39. B
40. B
41. A
42. A
43. B
44. D
45. D
46. A
47. E
48. A
49. D
50. E

## PROFICIENCY EXAM: UNIT III

1. A
2. C
3. E
4. D
5. C
6. D
7. D
8. B
9. A
10. D
11. B
12. D
13. B
14. C
15. D
16. B
17. E
18. B
19. D
20. C
21. A
22. E
23. A
24. D
25. B
26. C
27. A
28. A
29. D
30. C
31. E
32. A
33. D
34. A
35. E
36. C
37. B
38. A
39. D
40. A
41. A
42. C
43. D
44. E
45. D
46. D
47. D
48. B
49. E
50. A

# Copyrights and Acknowledgments

Figure 1.1: Reprinted, by permission, from Sobotta/Hammersen: HISTOLOGY: COLOR ATLAS OF MICROSCOPIC ANATOMY, 3rd Ed., © 1985, Urban & Schwarzenberg, Baltimore-Munich.

Figures 1.1, 1.2, and 3.24 are redrawn and modified, with permission, from Fawcett D: *Bloom and Fawcett: A Textbook of Histology,* ed 11, Philadelphia, W.B. Saunders Co, 1986.

Figures 1.3, 2.7, 2.14, 2.15, 2.17, 3.18, 3.25, 3.26, 3.27, 3.29, 3.39, 3.42, 3.43, and 3.45 are taken from *Clinical and Functional Histology for Medical Students* by Dr. R.S. Snell. Boston, Little Brown & Co, 1984. With permission.

Figure 1.4 is redrawn and modified, with permission, from Pysher TJ, Neustein HB: Ciliary Dysmorphology. *Perspectives in Pediatric Pathology* 1984: 8 (2), p. 102. Courtesy of Masson Publishing USA, Inc.

Figures 1.6, 2.3, 2.4, 2.5, 2.6, 2.10, 2.12, 3.7, 3.8, 3.9, 3.11, 3.13, 3.14, 3.20, 3.28, 3.30, 3.32, 3.33, 3.35, 3.41, 3.47, and 3.49 are redrawn, with permission, from Borysenko M, Beringer T: *Functional Histology,* ed 2. Boston, Little Brown & Co, 1984.

Figures 2.1, 2.2, 2.11, 3.31, and 3.52: Reproduced, with permission, from Junqueira LC, Carneiro J: *Basic Histology,* 4th ed. Copyright 1983 by Lange Medical Publications, Los Altos, California.

Figures 2.8 and 2.20 are redrawn and modified, with permission, from Leeson CR, Leeson TS, Paparo AA: *Textbook of Histology,* ed 5. Philadelphia, W.B. Saunders Co, 1985.

Figures 2.9, 3.6, 3.22, 3.36, 3.37, and 3.50 are redrawn, with permission, from Cormack DH: *Introduction to Histology,* Philadelphia, Lippincott, 1984.

Figures 2.13, 3.12, and 3.23 are redrawn and modified, with permission, from Ham AW, Cormack DH: *Histology,* ed 8. Philadelphia, Lippincott, 1979.

Figures 2.16, 2.18, and 2.19 are redrawn and modified, with permission, from Barr ML, Kiernan JA: *Human Nervous System: An Anatomical Viewpoint,* ed 4. Philadelphia, Lippincott, 1983.

Figure 3.1 is redrawn and modified, with permission, from Bacon RL, Niles NR: *Medical Histology.* New York, Springer-Verlag, 1983.

Figure 3.17: Redrawn by permission from Millard M: *Lung, Pleura and Mediastinum* in Anderson WAD, Kissane, JM (eds): *Pathology,* 7th edition. St. Louis, 1977, The C.V. Mosby Company.

Figure 3.21 is redrawn and modified, with permission, from Lentz TL: *Cell Fine Structure: An Atlas of Drawings of Whole-Cell Structure.* Philadelphia, W.B. Saunders Co, 1971.

Figure 3.46 from Noback CR, Demarest RJ: *The Human Nervous System.* Copyright 1975 by McGraw-Hill, Inc. As adapted from Dowling and Boycott, 1966, by Noback and Laemle in *The Primate's Brain.* Appleton-Century-Crofts, Inc., 1970.

Figure 3.51 is redrawn, with permission, from Elias H, Pauly JE: *Human Microanatomy,* ed 3. F.A. Davis Co, 1966.